PCOS

FOR

DUMMIES

by Gaynor Bussell and Sharon Perkins, RN

WILEY

John Wiley & Sons, Inc.

PCOS For Dummies®

Published by
John Wiley & Sons, Inc.
111 River St.
Hoboken, NJ 07030-5774
www.wiley.com

Copyright © 2011 by John Wiley & Sons, Inc., Hoboken, New Jersey

Published simultaneously in Canada

For general information on our other products and services, please contact our Customer Care Department within the U.S. at 877-762-2974, outside the U.S. at 317-572-3993, or fax 317-572-4002.

For technical support, please visit www.wiley.com/techsupport.

Wiley publishes in a variety of print and electronic formats and by print-on-demand. Some material included with standard print versions of this book may not be included in e-books or in print-on-demand. If this book refers to media such as a CD or DVD that is not included in the version you purchased, you may download this material at http://booksupport.wiley.com. For more information about Wiley products, visit www.wiley.com.

Library of Congress Control Number: 2011930314

ISBN 978-1-118-09865-3 (pbk); ISBN 978-1-118-12735-3 (ebk); ISBN 978-1-118-12736-0 (ebk); ISBN 978-1-118-12737-7 (ebk)

Manufactured in the United States of America

V10005128_101018

WILEY

About the Authors

Gaynor Bussell: Gaynor Bussell is a registered dietitian, a nutrition consultant, and a member of various professional nutrition organizations, including the Nutrition Society and the British Dietetic Association.

Gaynor began specializing in women's health after taking a short career break to have her two daughters. She worked as a women's health dietitian for over six years at University College Hospital in London, specializing particularly in PMS, menopause, preconception health, eating disorders, and, of course, PCOS. She also covered the osteoporosis clinic at this hospital. During this time, Gaynor became dietary advisor to a women's health charity.

Since then, Gaynor has worked at various women's health clinics, including those at Hammersmith and Queen Charlotte's. She was also the dietitian for a private residential eating disorders center. Gaynor continues to see private patients who have women's health issues and/or eating disorders. She also continues to work with various women's health organizations and charities, and writes and gives talks on various aspects of women's health.

Gaynor currently works as a consultant for the Food and Drink Federation (FDF), where her role includes acting as the interface on nutritional matters between industry and UK and EU authorities and sitting on a number of decision-making committees.

Sharon Perkins: Sharon Perkins is a registered nurse with over 20 years of experience, mostly in women's health and ophthalmology. She is also an online medical writer and author of seven *For Dummies* books, including *Infertility For Dummies, Osteoporosis For Dummies, Breastfeeding For Dummies, Endometriosis For Dummies, Healthy Aging For Dummies,* and *Dad's Guide to Pregnancy For Dummies* (all published by Wiley). She enjoys all her jobs equally but enjoys her three grandchildren, five children, two daughters-in-law, one son-in-law, family, and friends more! She lives in New Jersey but spends a lot of time gallivanting around the country and would live in Walt Disney World if she could.

Dedication

This is dedicated to all the women with PCOS we've gotten to know over the years.

Authors' Acknowledgments

Gaynor Bussell: Thanks to the excellent team at Wiley, in particular Rachael Chilvers and Alison Yates, who kept me encouraged and did not shout too much when deadlines were missed!

Thanks to my family: David and my two daughters, Sally and Jenny. Thanks guys about being good-natured and understanding about my "being on a roll" so that dinner didn't get served until 10 p.m., again!

Thanks to my work colleagues at the Food and Drink Federation who allowed me to take the time out to write the book and always took an interest in how things were coming along.

Finally, thanks to the team at Next Generation gym. You sorted out my mouse-strained shoulder and gave me excellent workout plans. It was great to go to you as a bolt hole when I needed to think, de-stress, and pound the life out of a treadmill!

Sharon Perkins: It's always fun to acknowledge all the people who take a book from idea to finished product. Many thanks to our editor, Elizabeth Kuball, who made this book easy from start to finish, and to Acquisitions Editor Erin Calligan Mooney for making it happen in the first place. Also, thanks to technical editor Josh Krotec, for jumping in when I needed him (again!). To all the behind-the-scenes people at Wiley, whose names I never learn but who make each book the best it can be, I'm very grateful.

Publisher's Acknowledgments

We're proud of this book; please send us your comments at http://dummies.custhelp.com. For other comments, please contact our Customer Care Department within the U.S. at 877-762-2974, outside the U.S. at 317-572-3993, or fax 317-572-4002.

Some of the people who helped bring this book to market include the following:

Acquisitions, Editorial, and Media Development

Project Editor: Elizabeth Kuball

Acquisitions Editor: Erin Calligan Mooney

Copy Editor: Elizabeth Kuball

Assistant Editor: David Lutton

Editorial Program Coordinator: Joe Niesen

Technical Editor:
Joseph W. Krotec, MD, FACOG

Senior Editorial Manager: Jennifer Ehrlich

Editorial Supervisor and Reprint Editor:
Carmen Krikorian

Editorial Assistants: Alexa Koschler

Art Coordinator: Alicia B. South

Cover Photos: iStockphoto.com/nkbimages

Cartoons: Rich Tennant
(www.the5thwave.com)

Composition Services

Project Coordinator: Katherine Crocker

Layout and Graphics: Corrie Socolovitch

Proofreaders:
BIM Indexing & Proofreading Services,
Dwight Ramsey

Indexer: Potomac Indexing, LLC

Illustrators: Kathryn Born,
Elizabeth Kurtzman

Publishing and Editorial for Consumer Dummies

    Kathleen Nebenhaus, Vice President and Executive Publisher

    David Palmer, Associate Publisher

    Kristin Ferguson-Wagstaffe, Product Development Director

Publishing for Technology Dummies

    Andy Cummings, Vice President and Publisher

Composition Services

    Debbie Stailey, Director of Composition Services

Contents at a Glance

Table of Contents

Introduction

*W*hen you're first diagnosed with polycystic ovary syndrome (PCOS), you may have a million questions about how this disorder will affect your life. No one wants a disease that doesn't have a cure! However, the good news is that you can, with work, keep your PCOS symptoms more or less completely at bay. This doesn't happen simply by taking a pill or two — you have to put in the effort yourself, and you aren't going to see results overnight. That's not a message that everyone likes to hear in today's instant-gratification society. The rewards are huge though — you get your life back, and you feel so much healthier that you don't *want* to return to your old lifestyle.

Put simply, you need to live a healthy life to keep PCOS under control. Lose any excess weight, get fit, tone up, and eat food that's going to give your body the biggest bang for the buck. In some cases, medications can help prevent complications and get your symptoms under control. All this doesn't need to be dull and boring: Not only can being physically active be fun, but it can literally change your life. Eating right gives you more energy for life and can taste surprisingly good, too.

For many women with PCOS, pregnancy is a huge concern. Getting pregnant may not be as easy for you as it is for some women, but this book gives you all the info you need on the help that's out there. If you need fertility treatments, we give you the basic rundown on what to expect.

About This Book

When you're first told that you have a particular medical condition, people come out of the woodwork to tell you third-hand stories about the experiences of friends and long-lost relatives. And, more than likely, everyone's advice contradicts the advice of the last person you talked to. You may have looked up PCOS online or leafed through a few books about it. You may even have read articles about it in popular magazines, or read about some celebrity who cured herself by eating nothing but peanut butter sandwiches. What's a girl to do when faced with the garden of misinformation, half-truths, and dire predictions about PCOS available 24/7 online and elsewhere?

This book gives you down-to-earth and up-to-date advice. It tells you what has worked and what hasn't for PCOS sufferers, and takes you through what you can be doing for yourself to help reduce your PCOS symptoms, as well as what medical treatments are available for PCOS. Being able to discuss your medical condition knowledgably with your doctor helps you to be a proactive patient.

And it does all this as a reference book — not something you have to read from beginning to end, but something you can dip into to find the information you need when you need it.

Conventions Used in This Book

We use the following conventions throughout this book to help keep things consistent and easy to understand:

- ✔ When we introduce a new term, we put it in *italics* and define it shortly thereafter, often in parentheses.

- ✔ All web addresses appear in monofont. *Note:* When this book was printed, some web addresses may have needed to break across two lines of text. If that happened, rest assured that we haven't put in any extra characters (such as hyphens) to indicate the break. So, when using one of these web addresses, just type in exactly what you see in this book, pretending as though the line break doesn't exist.

What You're Not to Read

If you want to get straight to the nitty-gritty, and extract all the vital bits as quickly as possible so you can make a start on what you need to do, you can skip the following information and still accomplish your goal:

- ✔ **Text in sidebars:** These gray boxes appear here and there throughout the book. They share anecdotes and observations, but they aren't essential reading.

- ✔ **Anything marked by a Technical Stuff icon:** This information pumps you with a few more technical facts or background about a particular subject, but it isn't essential reading if you don't want to know the why, just the how.

Of course, when you're ready (and have the time or curiosity to spare), remember that these pieces of info are well worth dipping into.

Foolish Assumptions

Every *For Dummies* book is written with a particular reader in mind, and this one is no exception. So, I made the following basic assumptions about you:

- You're not a doctor, so you don't have (or want) the technical understanding about the PCOS condition, but you are interested in getting a basic understanding of it.

- You have PCOS, and you want to know how to reduce your symptoms so that you can improve your quality of life.

- You're confused about the right dietary and exercise route to take to get you on track to reducing your symptoms.

- You're dissatisfied with quick fixes, fads, and wonder diets and treatments and need a realistic alternative that works.

- You want straight-talking, understandable information. You want to learn about possible complications and issues that women with PCOS face so you can deal with them intelligently, but you don't need to become an expert on PCOS.

- You want to get pregnant and have heard that pregnancy is difficult for women with PCOS. Rest assured, we address your pregnancy concerns in detail.

- You don't want to spend hours digging around for information, but you do want a one-stop shop that cuts to the chase but doesn't mislead you.

How This Book Is Organized

The great thing about *For Dummies* books is that you don't have to read them all the way through. You can simply turn to the bit you want — a chapter, a section, even just a paragraph. The table of contents and the index help you out. This section gives you an idea of what lies ahead.

Part 1: PCOS in a Nutshell

When you're initially diagnosed with any condition, the first order of business is getting a good enough understanding so that (1) you're not terrified or panicky and (2) you can make good decisions about how to take care of your health. So, in this part, we give you basic information about PCOS: what it is, what causes it, what symptoms may accompany it, what changes you can expect as you age, and — most important — how you can take control and manage it.

Part II: Taking Control of Your Symptoms

In this part, we talk about the underlying causes of PCOS so you know what you're dealing with. Then it's time to discuss all the nitty-gritty topics of everyday life — diet, exercise, medications, supplements, and keeping your mind and body balanced so you don't go over the edge dealing with it all.

Part III: Menstrual Cycles, Fertility, and Pregnancy

PCOS can really turn your hormonal life upside down, and your menstrual cycle and fertility can take a beating in the process. This part shows you how to turn your menstrual cycle right-side up again and discusses fertility issues that can loom large when you have PCOS. Last, we look at the effects of PCOS on pregnancy and give you tips on how to get pregnant, with or without medical help, and how to deliver a healthy baby at the end of it all.

Part IV: The Part of Tens

This part contains four chapters of ten tips each, which form a quick reference guide. Most of these tips are mentioned throughout the rest of the book, but this part brings them all together as a handy reference.

Here you find tips on the PCOS symptoms that you can diminish by using the advice in this book; discover how to distinguish the good diets from the bad; and identify ten superfoods you can incorporate into your diet to help reduce your PCOS symptoms. Finally, the last chapter lists ten sources of support and advice for people who have PCOS or have a close friend or relative with it.

Icons Used in This Book

Icons are a handy *For Dummies* way to catch your attention as you slide your eyes down the page. The icons come in several varieties, each with its own unique symbol and meaning.

Your understanding of the health and diet world may be riddled with myths or old wives' tales. Some of them may be based on truth, but most came from another planet and don't apply to human beings today. This symbol means that the myth has been exposed for what it is.

This symbol marks the place where you can find explanations of the terms used by nutrition experts.

This icon draws your attention to an important point to keep in mind when dealing with PCOS.

These details add to your understanding of PCOS. You can get on in life perfectly fine without them, so skip them if you want to, but try a few first — they may give you some facts that may help you to answer the questions on obscure quiz shows!

The Tip icon does exactly what it says — cherish these little nuggets because they're there to make your life a little easier.

This icon points to certain pitfalls or things that may actually harm you. Ignore at your peril!

Where to Go from Here

Where to go from here? Wherever you like, and you certainly don't need to read from cover to cover, unless you like to follow tradition! You can dive right in anywhere in the book, because each chapter (and even each section) delivers a complete message. The table of contents is detailed enough to help you pinpoint the topic you want to know about.

If you want to know more about exercising to achieve weight loss, go straight to Chapter 6. If pregnancy is foremost on your mind, jump in at Chapter 11. If you're really not sure where to start, read Chapter 1, which gives you all the basic information about PCOS and helps you decide which area you want to home in on first.

Part I
PCOS in a Nutshell

The 5th Wave
By Rich Tennant

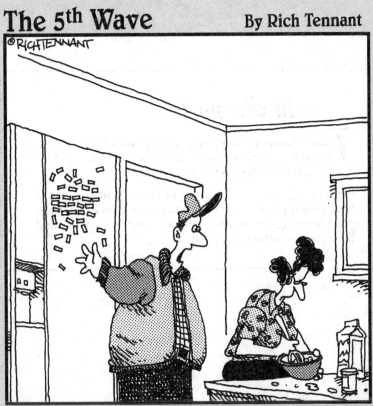

"It's been two months since your diagnosis, and I know you're reluctant to talk about it. But we've got to start discussing it in some way other than messages left on the refrigerator with these tiny word magnets."

In this part...

*T*his part gives you an overview of everything PCOS related and helps you identify whether you might have PCOS by listing all the symptoms.

In this part, you get some straight facts about your condition, how it plays out in your body, how it changes when you change (such as when you get older or heavier), and how you can start to tackle it.

Chapter 1

Sensible and Straightforward Solutions for a Difficult Condition

. . . .

In This Chapter

▶ Understanding PCOS and its symptoms

▶ Taking the initial steps when you think you may have PCOS

▶ Tackling PCOS through diet, exercise, and emotional well-being

▶ Looking at treatment options

▶ Working out what you can do to help yourself

. . . .

*T*his chapter is a great place to get on the right course if you suffer or suspect you suffer from PCOS, or if you have a friend, relative, or partner with the condition and you want a quick overview of the most important things you need to know about PCOS.

This chapter gives an overview of the entire book. In one chapter you get a feel for what PCOS really is and what its symptoms are. Just as important, you get an overview of treatments and lifestyle changes that are aimed at reducing the symptoms; many are things that you can do to help yourself.

Understanding PCOS

PCOS is the most common ovarian function disorder in pre-menopausal women. Yet, until recently, it was one of the least-understood conditions. Research into the causes and symptoms of PCOS has shown it to have consequences more far-reaching than the obvious physical symptoms; the long-term effects extend into menopause and beyond.

Defining the condition

According to the American Society for Reproductive Medicine, PCOS is defined as having any two of the following signs and symptoms:

- ✔ *Oligo-ovulation* (irregular ovulation) or *anovulation* (a complete lack of ovulation)
- ✔ Clinical or biochemical signs of high *androgen* (male hormone) levels
- ✔ Polycystic ovaries, which means many small cysts on the ovaries (normal ovaries have five or six follicles, whereas polycystic ovaries have ten or more)

The hormones involved in controlling periods and, ultimately, reproduction, are produced in the pituitary gland, located in the brain. In women with PCOS, two of these hormones — luteinizing hormone (LH) and follicle stimulating hormone (FSH) — are produced in abnormal proportions. The imbalance of these two hormones prevents the follicles in the ovary from developing properly: The follicles tend to remain small and don't mature enough to release an egg. As a result, a string of small follicles, or cysts, form on the ovary, giving rise to the characteristic polycystic ovary that gives the disorder its name.

Polycystic ovaries alone are not enough to diagnose PCOS. If the symptoms of PCOS do develop, that marks the change from simply having symptom-free polycystic ovaries to having PCOS. Around 20 percent of women have polycystic ovaries but no symptoms of PCOS.

PCOS statistics

The rates of PCOS appear to be increasing. Increasing rates of PCOS are most likely to be related to the rise in obesity rates in the United States. Around 68 percent of all adults in the United States are now overweight or obese, and, even more alarming, 20 percent of children ages 6 to 11 and 18 percent of teens are overweight. The potential increase in overweight even in children could herald the development of even more women developing PCOS in the future.

Chew on these PCOS statistics for more on how this disorders affects women of nearly all ages:

- ✔ Around 5 million American women have PCOS.
- ✔ PCOS can start in girls as young as age 11.
- ✔ About 5 percent to 10 percent of American women have PCOS.

It's in the genes

Researchers in the United States studied 215 mothers of women with PCOS and compared them with mothers of women who didn't have PCOS. Results showed that mothers of women with PCOS themselves had some of the symptoms of PCOS, including high cholesterol levels, insulin resistance, and other metabolic abnormalities associated with PCOS.

In addition, a high proportion of these mothers who had daughters with PCOS reported that they had had menstrual irregularities. Those mothers who had reported the menstrual problems had higher male hormone levels than those who hadn't reported irregularities.

All this points to the fact that the mothers of daughters with PCOS had a much higher incidence of PCOS symptoms than mothers of non-PCOS daughters. It seemed that whether the mothers had been diagnosed with PCOS or not, a genetic tendency was definitely present.

Knowing you're at risk

The exact cause of PCOS is unclear, but certain conditions do predispose women to developing it:

- ✔ **Being obese, especially if obesity began before puberty:** Overweight that develops before puberty appears to increase male androgen levels.

- ✔ **Elevated insulin levels:** High insulin levels stimulate increased male hormone production.

- ✔ **Genetics:** You're at increased risk if your mother or sister has the condition or if your father has female family members with PCOS.

Here are the stats showing the genetic tendency toward PCOS (you can read more about the link in the sidebar "It's in the genes"):

- ✔ Thirty-five percent of PCOS sufferers inherit the disorder from their mother.

- ✔ Thirty-five percent of PCOS sufferers inherit the disorder from their father's side of the family.

- ✔ Fifty percent of PCOS sufferers have female relatives with PCOS on both sides of their family.

✔ In one study, 77 percent of women with PCOS had a close relative with PCOS; 50 percent had a mother or sister with the disorder and 25 percent had a maternal or paternal aunt with PCOS.

A single gene responsible for PCOS has not been found. Developing PCOS may be a complex issue with genetic, environmental, and lifestyle components, such as early diet.

Identifying the symptoms

The symptoms of PCOS vary from woman to woman and can be present in any combination. They also can change over time, so if you have PCOS, your symptoms are likely to be different from someone else you know with PCOS.

The most common PCOS symptoms include the following:

✔ **Weight gain, especially around the tummy:** Turn to Chapter 2 for more on the causes and effects of weight gain in women with PCOS and check out Chapter 5 for help with losing weight.

✔ **Increased hairiness on the face and other regions (called *hirsutism*):** Excess *androgens* (male hormones) cause these symptoms. We talk more about the effects and treatments of excess hair where you don't want it in Chapter 2.

✔ **Male pattern baldness or thinning hair:** This symptom, another side effect of increased male hormones, is also addressed in more detail in Chapter 2.

✔ **Oily skin with acne:** This is another side effect of androgen production. We cover it in greater detail in Chapter 2.

✔ **Absent or irregular menstrual cycles:** This condition leads to infertility. The issues of the menstrual cycle are discussed in detail in Chapter 10. Ways to improve fertility are found in Chapter 11.

✔ **Insulin resistance:** Being insulin resistant means your body can't use insulin efficiently. This leads to high circulating blood levels of insulin (called *hyperinsulinemia*). High levels of insulin in the blood may cause PCOS symptoms to worsen gradually. Being diagnosed with insulin resistance also increases your chances of having PCOS. See Chapter 3 for an in-depth discussion of insulin resistance and its role in PCOS.

Taking Your First Steps toward Living with PCOS

If you suspect you have PCOS, your first reaction may be panic, followed by anger or depression. Without proper care, PCOS can impact nearly every aspect of your life, so fear, anxiety, and worry are normal reactions — but don't hold onto them for too long! Be proactive in your care by taking positive steps toward improving your health and finding a medical care partner who can guide you on the way.

But also remember, first and foremost, that this is *your* medical condition and *your* life. No one has more motivation or more to gain from getting PCOS under control than you do. Take these first steps:

- **Find a knowledgeable medical practitioner.** This may or may not be your current family doctor or gynecologist. Finding someone who has a real interest in PCOS may take some sleuthing and involvement in support groups (group members normally have the inside track on who's good at treating the condition), which leads to the next step. . . .

- **Get involved with a support group.** If there are support groups in your area, tap into their resources, because they're your best source for competent and concerned medical care. If you have no local support groups, connect with people online. Chapter 16 has a list of resources on PCOS, including helpful websites if there are no active groups in your area or you're not the joining type.

- **Do your research.** Some practitioners may not be up on the latest info on PCOS, so make sure *you* are. Read everything you can find online, particularly from reputable organizations like the American Congress of Obstetricians and Gynecologists (www.acog.org), Mayo Clinic (www.mayoclinic.com), or the Polycystic Ovarian Syndrome Association (www.pcosupport.org). Take with a grain of salt anything you read on lesser-known sites — the Internet is home to a number of charlatans with questionable medical practices. Check out applicable books from your library, but pay attention to the publication dates to make sure you're getting the latest info. Invest in a few well-recommended books, including this one!

- **Stay active and involved with life.** PCOS isn't life-threatening, but it can cause dangerous complications if it gets out of control. Letting PCOS become your whole life is as unproductive as ignoring it completely.

✔ **Find ways to cope with stress.** After you're diagnosed, it can be a relief to know that the symptoms aren't just in your mind. But then you're left with the stress of knowing that you have to cope with a long-term condition. Empower yourself by knowing what PCOS is and what you can do about it so that you're in control — this strategy can help to lessen the emotional frustrations.

The Three-Pronged Attack

Unfortunately, no cure exists for PCOS, but you can control the symptoms so that the effect of PCOS on your body is minimal. To decrease symptoms of PCOS, you need to tackle the following issues:

✔ **Improving insulin sensitivity:** This improvement prevents the whole cascade of later problems, such as developing type 2 diabetes and abnormal blood fat levels, which can give rise to heart disease. (See Chapter 3 for the details on how insulin resistance develops and how it causes many of the symptoms associated with PCOS.)

✔ **Restoring normal ovulation, which helps restore normal fertility:** Part III tells you how to improve menstrual symptoms and increase your chances of getting pregnant.

✔ **Stopping androgen levels in the blood from rising.**

Although medications may help, you also can do your part by mounting a three-pronged attack using the following tools at your disposal:

✔ **Diet:** Follow a low-glycemic-index diet. See Chapter 4 for information on the *glycemic index* (a way of categorizing foods by their effect on your blood glucose levels) and how the glycemic index affects PCOS symptoms.

✔ **Exercise:** Strive to be more physically active on a day-to-day basis and throughout the day. Exercise not only improves mood but increases weight loss.

✔ **Emotional well-being:** If you lack motivation or are moody and/or depressed, try some techniques for mood lifting and motivation. Maintaining a positive attitude can have a positive effect on your physical as well as your mental health.

 Even if you're at a normal weight, research has shown that if you have PCOS, you still have a tendency to have higher blood concentrations of insulin compared to women without PCOS of the same weight. So, eating a low-GI, balanced diet and being physically active is important, even if you don't have a weight problem.

Treatment should be tailored to you and the symptoms you're experiencing, but it should also take into consideration whether you're aiming to get pregnant. If you're not planning on having a baby just yet, treatment needs to focus on:

- Correcting abnormal hormone levels

- Losing weight (or maintaining a healthy weight if you aren't overweight)

- Managing cosmetic concerns (such as increased hairiness where you don't want hair, and the loss of hair on your head where you do want it)

If you're hoping to get pregnant, treatment needs to focus on:

- Losing weight, because a healthy diet with increased physical activity allows more efficient use of insulin and decreases blood glucose levels and may help you to ovulate more regularly

- Promoting ovulation with ovulation-induction medications

Maximizing your health before you conceive and normalizing blood glucose and blood insulin levels help ensure that, if you do conceive, there's less risk of miscarrying or having a baby that develops problems. (See Chapter 12 for more on the risks of pregnancy with PCOS.)

Diet under the spotlight

The high insulin level commonly found in PCOS sufferers is to blame for the tendency to gain weight and the inability to lose it. That's why, when you have PCOS, your diet is of vital importance because you have to balance several factors: calorie intake (to avoid excess weight gain), carbohydrate intake (to stabilize blood sugars), and so on.

A PCOS-friendly diet helps you to

- Lose weight to get to a healthy weight, or to maintain a healthy weight

- Reduce insulin resistance and the risk of developing type 2 diabetes

- Reduce the risk of cardiovascular disease

- Ensure a balanced and nutritionally adequate dietary intake

For detailed information on the low-GI diet and how to lose weight successfully, head to Chapters 4 and 5.

Diets to avoid

Avoid diets that restrict the intake of certain groups of foods or ban them completely. Also avoid diets that advocate you take certain supplements. Such diets are likely to be unbalanced. Low-carb diets are often advocated in popular books and websites for PCOS. These diets aren't recommended by many doctors and dietitians because they:

✔ **Are high in fat:** A high-fat diet may raise your cholesterol level, putting you at a higher risk of heart disease. Several studies, however, show that low-carb diets lower cholesterol in some people.

✔ **Tend to be high in protein:** A high-protein diet may put you at a higher risk of kidney problems, especially if you already have diabetes, which can cause kidney damage.

✔ **Cause you to produce more ketones from the breakdown of fats:** Ketogenic diets are not recommended in pregnancy; high ketone levels in the blood could have damaging effects on the fetus.

Getting physical

The good news about getting more active is that it offers huge benefits to symptom reduction in PCOS. The benefits extend well beyond PCOS and into many other areas, from cancer prevention to improving your mental state. Chapter 8 tells you everything you need to know about the benefits of exercising, including different ways to exercise and how to vary your routine.

Benefits of exercise

The reasons to exercise if you have PCOS (and for general health) include the following:

✔ **To help maintain weight loss and allow you to have a few more calories while on a weight-loss diet:** The ideal combination is to lose weight by following a sensible weight-control diet along with a minimum of half an hour of physical activity a day.

✔ **To improve the relative amount of muscle to fat as well as overall body shape.**

✔ **To improve insulin sensitivity.**

✔ **To increase the levels of high-density lipoprotein (HDL), or "good" cholesterol, in the blood.**

✔ **To reduce blood pressure.**

✔ To decrease your risk of developing heart disease and diabetes.

✔ To improve bone density, reducing your risk of developing osteoporosis.

✔ To improve your psychological health, such as self-confidence, well-being, and self-image.

 To maximize the advantages of doing exercise, you need to combine aerobic exercise (which causes you to get a bit breathless) with some resistance training (such as lifting weights) and some stretching and flexibility work to maintain strain-free movement. Chapter 6 explains what you need to know.

Tips for exercising success

 There's a high dropout rate among people who take up exercise. To avoid this, plan ahead and keep a few things in mind:

✔ **Don't be too ambitious, or you'll never keep it up.** Instead of swearing that you'll swim for 30 minutes, run for 30 minutes, and bike for 30 minutes every day, shoot for something manageable, like a 30-minute walk.

✔ **Plan to do a form of exercise that fits into your lifestyle and that you enjoy doing.** If getting to a gym is difficult for you, choose an exercise you can do at home. When in doubt, opt for walking — you can do that anywhere, and you don't need anything other than a good pair of shoes.

✔ **If you don't have time to exercise — and who ever does, unless they're motivated enough to make time for it? — incorporate exercise into your daily routine.** For example, if you normally stop in at the grocery store to pick up a few things every day, think about walking or even bicycling there instead.

 The amount of moving about you do throughout the day is as important as any formal exercise session you undertake. So, think about how you can build in more activity throughout the day (take the stairs instead of the elevator, park far away from the mall entrance, and so on).

Looking after the inside

Knowing the wonderful results that you can achieve by diet and exercise is fine, but if an overload of stress, anxiety, or depression are preventing you from following through, having an encyclopedic knowledge of PCOS isn't going to do you a lot of good. In order to be able to act on your knowledge about what you should do, you need to feel empowered with the knowledge that you understand your condition, are ready to take action, and are on a fairly even keel, emotionally speaking.

An important key to getting well is to treat yourself kindly. Recognize that PCOS is a major stressor in your life and give yourself permission to work through the feelings associated with it. To diminish the symptoms associated with PCOS, you must also recognize the emotional effects of PCOS, accept them, and learn to deal with them.

PCOS often leads to feelings of anxiety, low self-esteem, and loss of control. The emotional effects of PCOS can start in the teenage years when the symptoms such as weight problems, excess facial or body hair, and acne, start to emerge. To make matters worse, the journey to a diagnosis can be long and painful.

Chapter 9 explains in more detail the effects of PCOS on your emotional well-being and offers strategies and advice on how to avoid or ameliorate the most common emotional pitfalls.

Trying Medications, Supplements, and More

Paying attention to your diet, your exercise levels, and your emotional health are things that you can do yourself, with a bit of support from friends, family, and some relevant experts such as personal trainers and dietitians. However, sometimes this just isn't enough and you have to get extra support, as outlined in the following sections.

Medications

Even if you get to work on the diet, exercise, and motivational advice in this book, your doctor may feel you also need some medication to help reduce your symptoms. This is especially important if you're at risk of developing other diseases such as diabetes, heart disease, or possibly even *endometrial cancer* (cancer of the uterine lining). See Chapter 7 for a rundown of different medications and their potential benefits.

Only take medication that is prescribed by your doctor or specialist especially for you.

Depending on your symptoms, medications can play an important part in your PCOS treatment. If you're having trouble getting pregnant, medications often become a necessity. Medications also can help with hair loss and acne as well as insulin resistance, which can decrease your chance of developing diabetes, as well as long-term complications such as high cholesterol and heart disease. Chapter 7 is loaded with information on the types of medications used to treat PCOS.

Supplements and herbals

When you read up on PCOS, you find that a whole plethora of herbal remedies and supplements are recommended for PCOS. Go to Chapter 8 for more information about supplements and herbals.

Be wary of advice you hear, especially from unproven sources. Supplements and herbal remedies can be harmful, especially if you decide to take them without the backing of a professional, medically qualified practitioner. Before you take any herbal or supplement, consult your doctor.

Alternative therapies

Natural remedies should be tried only if you follow the advice of an experienced, qualified practitioner with an interest in women's health, including fertility. At present, no clinical trials have been completed on alternative therapies in this area.

However, you can try some treatments that may help you to relax and that should be relatively safe, including acupuncture, massage, and reflexology. Chapter 8 discusses alternative therapies — both good and bad.

What about surgery?

Surgery is rarely used to treat PCOS. In some cases, however, a technique known as *ovarian drilling* may help women who are trying to get pregnant but who don't respond to medications given to regulate menstrual cycles and start ovulation. During this procedure, a doctor punctures a small hole in the ovary with an electric needle or laser that destroys part of the ovary.

Ovarian drilling can help decrease male hormone levels by reducing the number of cells producing those hormones, but the effect is usually short-lived and the procedure can cause scarring in the ovary and negatively affect fertility, which is why it's used only as a last resort.

Living a Lifetime with PCOS

Unfortunately, menstrual irregularities and the metabolic symptoms (such as insulin resistance and abnormal blood fat levels) of PCOS seem to be inherited and can cause diseases that persist throughout life. Also, unfortunately, neither the removal of ovaries nor going through menopause seems to eliminate the symptoms. However, you can look for a light at the end of the tunnel, and that is the fact that by adopting a healthy lifestyle you can reduce most symptoms to insignificant levels.

No cure exists for PCOS, but in many cases symptoms can be controlled. Treatment involves breaking the vicious cycle of insulin resistance and overweight, which leads to even higher insulin levels and triggers worsening PCOS symptoms. Remember, too, that not all women with PCOS are obese or even overweight — it's possible to have PCOS symptoms even when you're at a normal weight.

If you know you have PCOS in your family, one way to prevent it from developing in the first place or to minimize its effects is to stay within the right weight range. This can be measured by a ratio called the body mass index (BMI). To figure your BMI, go to www.nhlbisupport.com/bmi. (Chapter 5 has more information on BMI.)

Waist circumference is another way of checking how much fat you're carrying, particularly in the danger area around the middle. You're in the danger zone (as a woman) if your waist circumference is more than 31½ inches. See Chapter 5 for more on this and other weighty issues of PCOS.

Monitoring mood and motivation

Vicious cycles are common in PCOS. Getting into shape and reducing the symptoms can seem such an uphill struggle that it may seem easier just to give up. But in giving up, you feel more and more depressed and believe that extreme actions are required. However, extreme actions just set you up for failure again, and the circle continues.

To offset a complete relapse, keep the following in mind:

✔ **Tripping up from time to time is inevitable.** When it happens, pick yourself up and set yourself back on the road.

✔ **Start gradually.** Maybe begin with a ten-minute walk every day — everybody has ten minutes to spare, right? — and work your way up gradually to your goal. Adding a minute to your walk every few days won't seem that hard. And before you know it, you'll be walking 30 minutes or more!

✔ **Make sure that the changes can be incorporated easily into your lifestyle and that you can keep them up long term.**

✔ **Set yourself smaller mini goals along the way.** Reward yourself with something other than food (maybe a massage or a day at the spa) each time you achieve a mini goal.

Keep a food diary and an exercise diary. If keeping a diary permanently is too much, just fill it in for a week or two initially, and then from time to time when you feel your resolve is slacking. Keep track of your moods, too. A diary can remind you what you were doing when things were going well, but it also can help bring to light problems when things aren't going so well.

Avoiding eating disorders

With so much emphasis placed on staying at a normal weight if you have PCOS, it's inevitable that some women fall into the pattern of thinking that if a little weight loss is good, a lot if better. This belief can lead to eating disorders.

If you have a distorted pattern of thinking about and behaving around food, you may have an eating disorder. If you have an eating disorder, you'll also have a preoccupation and/or obsession with food, and your eating (or lack of eating) is likely to be out of control.

Any eating disorder requires professional help. Acknowledging what the triggers are to this behavior is important — they're frequently mood-based, especially feelings of low self-esteem.

Chapter 2

Knowing You Have PCOS

*I*f you have PCOS, you have the most common hormonal and reproductive problem affecting women of childbearing age. In recent years, it has become apparent that PCOS is much more common than was previously realized.

In the past, only women with the most severe symptoms were acknowledged to have the condition that is now known as PCOS. Nowadays, with much more advanced diagnostic tools (such as ultrasound) being available, doctors are better at recognizing the condition, even if the symptoms are only mild.

Previously, the condition was known as polycystic ovarian disease or Stein-Leventhal syndrome, after the two doctors who discovered it in the 1930s.

This chapter spells out how you can recognize if you have PCOS by exploring the physical, emotional, and hidden symptoms of PCOS. It also looks at how you or your doctor can spot PCOS and touches on how to cope with PCOS through your life stages.

Recognizing Common Symptoms and Side Effects of PCOS

To judge by the name, you would think that the most important symptom of PCOS was multiple cysts on the ovaries (sometimes described as a "string of pearls"). These cysts are immature *follicles,* the egg-containing structures in the ovary, one of which should grow monthly to *ovulate* (release an egg). The cysts themselves are harmless, but they're a symptom of the hormonal issues that often cause infertility in women with PCOS. PCOS is also accompanied by a host of other symptoms. (The word *syndrome* actually means "a group of symptoms.") The following sections outline the obvious and not-so-obvious symptoms of PCOS.

You and your PCOS are unique. Quite a few different symptoms occur with PCOS, but your combination of symptoms probably differs from someone else's symptom profile. Some symptoms are more common than others — namely, weight gain (especially around the middle), skin problems, hairiness, and a tendency toward diabetes and infertility.

Because many of the symptoms of PCOS don't affect the way you look, other people may not understand why you're not up to doing things or why you don't feel well. Other symptoms, like weight gain, are all too visible. The situation isn't all doom and gloom, though — these symptoms can start to lessen as you act on the advice in this book.

Hormonal effects

As a PCOS sufferer, you're more likely to have higher-than-normal levels of androgens wreaking havoc around your body. (*Androgens* are male hormones — the best known being testosterone — which all women produce in their ovaries.) The abnormal level of these male hormones, along with other hormonal disruption, is responsible for the period problems you may be experiencing.

Period problems

Not all women with PCOS have problems with their period. If you don't, consider yourself to be one of the lucky 20 percent of women with PCOS who have perfectly normal menstrual cycles. In PCOS, your period may be

✔ Absent altogether, known medically as *amenorrhea*

✔ Irregular, known medically as *oligomenorrhea*

✔ Heavy, known medically as *menorrhagia*

✔ Longer than normal, lasting for a more than a week

See Chapter 10 for more detail on the effects of PCOS on menstrual periods.

Hot flashes

Hot flashes, another sign of hormonal imbalance, are normally associated with menopause, but they can occur in PCOS, too. Hot flashes themselves don't cause any harm, but they are a nuisance and can disturb your sleep. Hot flashes are characterized by

- ✔ Rapid heart beat
- ✔ Rise in body temperature
- ✔ Clammy palms
- ✔ Sweating

Endometrial cancer

The lining of the uterus, known as the *endometrium,* varies in thickness throughout a normal monthly menstrual cycle. At the start of a normal menstrual cycle, the lining, which is normally thin, builds up in preparation for the implanting of a fertilized egg. However, if the egg is not fertilized, this extra lining is shed in a normal menstrual period.

Often, in PCOS, no egg is released, but the lining of the uterus still builds up under the influence of estrogen. However, because ovulation never happens, this lining is never shed but keeps building up. Known as *endometrial hyperplasia,* this condition can increase the risk of developing endometrial cancer, although even in PCOS, this cancer is not very common.

Restoring a normal menstrual cycle is important, not only for restoring fertility but also so that the risk of developing endometrial cancer is reduced. See Chapter 10 for more on the risk of endometrial cancer in PCOS.

Endometriosis

Having both PCOS and endometriosis is not uncommon, but no one really knows whether the two conditions are linked.

Endometriosis is a condition in which tissue that is similar to the lining of the uterus grows outside the uterus. The most common sites for endometriosis to develop are the pelvis, on the ovaries, and on the bowel. These endometrial growths react to estrogen just like the endometrium in the uterus. The tissues swell and then become painful during the month when the uterine lining would be building up. The endometrial tissue then bleeds when a normal period is due. Scarring can occur in the areas where bleeding occurs repeatedly.

If you have PCOS, you tend to have a lot of estrogen in your system and very little progesterone. Estrogen normally builds up the uterine lining, and progesterone causes changes that enable it to accept an embryo. When progesterone is withdrawn, it triggers the monthly bleed. In PCOS, there is no ovulation and, thus, no progesterone — and being in a mode of continual buildup of uterine tissue without the effects of progesterone is just what you don't need if you have endometriosis, because this is likely to make the condition worse.

Fertility problems

Your PCOS may first have been diagnosed because you were trying to conceive but couldn't. When an ovary doesn't produce an egg, the result is infertility. An egg is not produced because the levels of hormones are insufficient to mature an egg in the ovary, so it doesn't get released.

Infertility usually happens when PCOS becomes quite advanced. Around 90 percent to 95 percent of women attending infertility clinics due to lack of ovulation have PCOS. You can help to restore your fertility by adopting the lifestyle changes outlined in this book. See Part III for more on the menstrual cycle, fertility treatments that can help you, and the risks of pregnancy if you have PCOS.

The battle of the bulge

You have a 50 percent chance of being overweight if you have PCOS (but that also means you have a 50 percent chance of *not* being overweight). Insulin resistance and the increased levels of male hormones that occur in PCOS are believed to be the main causes of weight gain, which occurs particularly around the middle. (See Chapter 5 for ways to battle the plague of weight gain in PCOS.) Not being able to control weight gain is often the most distressing symptom of PCOS.

The elevated levels of glucose in your bloodstream, which usually occur after you eat a carbohydrate-containing meal, trigger the pancreas to release insulin, which allows the cells in the body (such as muscle cells) to absorb the glucose. If you're *insulin resistant* (a common condition in PCOS), excessive amounts of free-floating glucose remain in the bloodstream because it can't properly enter the cells. This excess amount is eventually sent to the liver, where it is converted to excess body fat.

The symptoms of PCOS are more severe if you gain a lot of weight; as you lose weight, the symptoms diminish. If you're an overweight woman with PCOS, even a modest weight loss of 5 percent leads to

✔ A decrease in your insulin level

✔ An improvement in your menstrual cycle (or acts as a trigger for it to start again)

✔ Reduced testosterone levels, leading to reductions in *hirsutism* (hairiness) and acne

Fatigue and exhaustion

Feelings of exhaustion and fatigue are common in PCOS. Many factors, both physical and psychological, can lead to fatigue.

 With PCOS, the root cause of the feeling of tiredness and exhaustion is resistance to insulin, which makes your body turn the carbohydrates you eat into fat rather than a fuel source for energy. So, at the same time as you're gaining more and more weight, you also feel more and more tired. Also, blood sugars may dip quite low overnight if you suffer from PCOS, giving rise to fatigue the next day.

Several other causes can also contribute to feeling worn out and exhausted:

✔ **Lack of sleep** is common in PCOS and affects how awake you feel the next day. The hormonal fluctuations underlying PCOS can mean that you experience difficulties in getting a full night's sleep. Worry and frustration associated with having PCOS also may be contributing to any rough nights you're experiencing.

✔ The **stress and anxiety** brought about by having PCOS can lead to developing fatigue.

✔ **Depression,** which can occur in PCOS, also can cause feelings of tiredness.

✔ Because of **insulin resistance,** the muscles in your body can't always get enough glucose to convert to energy, which results in physical tiredness. Also, blood sugars can sometimes suddenly drop quite low, which also can result in feelings of fatigue and shakiness.

✔ Developing full-blown **type 2 diabetes,** something you're at greater risk of with PCOS, can make you feel tired, especially if you aren't keeping it under control.

✔ If, in an attempt to lose weight, you put yourself on **a diet that's too strict or restricts you from eating certain foods,** you lack energy. If you want to lose weight for your PCOS, choose a balanced, low-GI diet of around 1,500 calories per day, as advocated in this book, to give you more zing and not less!

✔ **Medications** to relieve PCOS can sometimes cause fatigue.

✔ If you have very heavy periods (which can happen sometimes if you have PCOS), you may have **iron-deficiency anemia,** which can cause fatigue.

If you feel tired all the time, discuss this fatigue with your doctor. She can check out any obvious causes, and may alter your medication.

 If you follow a healthy, low-GI, balanced diet, which includes a wide variety of foods and is not too calorie restrictive, you can help offset fatigue. You need to couple this diet with some regular physical activity. When you're tired, exercise may be the last thing you want to do, but get started, and you'll probably find that exercise actually boosts your energy levels, as long as you don't overdo it.

Digestive disorders

Many women with PCOS have digestive problems, especially constipation and irritable bowel syndrome (IBS). The reason why is not clear, but it can be linked to the fact that you may have a lowered metabolic rate after a meal, which may result in food taking longer to digest and not being digested efficiently.

In the same way that fluctuating hormone levels may lead to nausea in pregnancy and also during PMS, the altered hormone levels in PCOS can give rise to nausea. Abdominal pain and perpetual hunger are also common digestive symptoms of PCOS.

Insulin resistance

If you have PCOS, you may be told that you have insulin resistance. Insulin resistance, with the resultant high level of circulating insulin, is very common in PCOS. This condition is due to the muscles becoming resistant to the action of insulin, so that more insulin has to be pumped out to have any effect. Insulin resistance is more likely if you gain weight.

One of insulin's functions in your body is to help your cells take up glucose, which is used to create energy. If you're insulin resistant, not only do you end up feeling tired and lacking in energy, but also, because your cells can't utilize glucose in the blood, blood sugar levels rise, resulting in type 2 diabetes. Type 2 diabetes is known as a silent but deadly condition because its symptoms can go unnoticed for many years, by which time damage to the eyes and kidneys may have occurred and risk factors for heart disease increased. (Chapter 3 has much more on the effects of insulin resistance.)

Insulin resistance also leads to the development of abnormal levels of fats in the blood with rising levels of harmful cholesterol, increasing your chances of having heart disease or a stroke.

Insulin resistance is the root of most symptoms in PCOS. When insulin resistance is present, normal amounts of insulin are insufficient to bring down blood glucose levels, which are a result of consuming carbohydrates. Your pancreas has to make even more insulin to compensate, which leads to a rise in the amount of insulin circulating through your body. High insulin levels mean that

- ✔ Your body stores more fat, resulting in weight gain.

- ✔ Your ovaries produce more testosterone, which has an adverse effect on the reproductive hormones that control the formation of follicles in the ovary. The result is that your menstrual cycle may become irregular or your periods may even stop altogether.

- ✔ Extra testosterone causes more free testosterone to circulate in your body, causing acne and hirsutism.

Type 2 diabetes

Type 2 diabetes is a common complication of high insulin levels and insulin resistance in PCOS. The two types of diabetes are

- ✔ **Type 1:** Normally occurs in childhood or in a young person. The pancreas simply stops producing insulin altogether, possibly as part of an autoimmune reaction, so injections of insulin must be given for the rest of the person's life.

- ✔ **Type 2:** Type 2 diabetes (which usually develops in adults but increasingly is showing up in teens and children as the incidence of overweight in the United States continues to burgeon out of control) is normally preceded by insulin resistance. The pancreas is still capable of producing insulin, and it does so in increasing amounts, but the body is resistant to it. This can happen when someone gains too much weight. Eventually, if weight remains high or continues to increase, the body may give up producing insulin altogether, so like its type 1 cousin, insulin may be required in order to keep blood sugar levels at a controlled level.

More often, type 2 diabetes is managed by medications that lower insulin resistance. (See Chapter 7 for a list of medications used to treat type 2 diabetes.) Both type 1 and type 2 diabetes can cause similar long-term damage to the body if blood sugars are not controlled sufficiently. The effects include heart disease, kidney damage, gangrene, and blindness. See Chapter 3 for more about diabetes and its relationship to insulin resistance.

Metabolic syndrome

Metabolic syndrome (also known as syndrome X) is a cluster of conditions — including obesity, high blood sugar, high blood pressure, and high levels of harmful blood fats — that often occur together, putting you at an increased risk of getting heart disease and type 2 diabetes.

If you have PCOS, you have an elevenfold increased risk of developing metabolic syndrome; around 45 percent of women with PCOS have metabolic syndrome. (Fortunately, your risk of getting it decreases if you put into practice some of the advice in this book!). The diagnosis of metabolic syndrome is made when you have at least three of the following going on in your body:

- ✓ Abdominal obesity (excessive fat tissue in and around the abdomen).

- ✓ Abnormal blood fat levels, which includes high triglycerides, low HDL cholesterol ("good" cholesterol), and high LDL cholesterol ("bad" cholesterol). These together cause plaque buildups in the artery walls.

- ✓ High blood pressure.

- ✓ Insulin resistance, where the body can't properly use insulin and more is pumped out to compensate.

- ✓ An increase in certain substances in the blood that increase the likelihood of blood clots.

- ✓ A rise in substances in the blood (such as C-reactive protein) that cause inflammation, leading to an increased risk of damage to the artery walls and an increased risk of cardiovascular disease.

With PCOS, you're more likely to have metabolic syndrome if you gain a lot of weight or your periods have stopped (even though you aren't menopausal).

PCOS is a condition that can be relieved by breaking the vicious cycle of weight gain, which leads to worsening of symptoms and the development of new symptoms. By losing weight, you can reverse the symptoms of metabolic syndrome and regain your periods. Gaining weight leads to an increasing likelihood of your periods stopping, a worsening of metabolic syndrome, and the developing of full-blown diabetes.

Skin changes

You may develop *skin tags* (small pieces of skin that form on the neck, groin, or armpits). Skin tags are annoying and sometimes unsightly growths that can bleed if they're irritated by clothes rubbing against them. They can be removed easily by a dermatologist.

You also may develop darkened skin areas on the back of the neck, in the armpits, or under the breasts. The medical term for this condition is *acanthosis nigricans*. Acanthosis nigricans is not exclusive to PCOS; a number of medical conditions can cause the darkened, thick, velvety patches. Over half of adults who weigh twice as much as they should have acanthosis nigricans. Insulin resistance is the most common cause of acanthosis nigricans. Dark-skinned women are more likely than fair-skinned women to develop this disorder. Reducing insulin resistance by losing weight will help; there are no other specific treatments.

Acne and oily skin

Acne as a teenager is bad enough, but having it as a full-grown adult is even worse. Acne, a common symptom of PCOS, is an inflammatory skin disorder that involves interactions between hormones, hair, *sebaceous* (oil-secreting) glands, and bacteria. High androgen levels can lead to acne on your face, chest, or back. The skin's sebaceous glands are stimulated to overproduce an oily substance called *sebum* and this overproduction gives rise to acne.

The acne brought about by PCOS can be mild or severe, but it's likely to be worse if you're overweight. This is because the heavier you are, the more likely you are to have worsening insulin resistance, which causes a rise in the level of androgens. One particular androgen, a metabolite of testosterone called DHT (dihydrotestosterone), stimulates the production of oil in the sebaceous glands of the skin, which eventually can lead to clogged glands or pores.

Clogged pores, which can't release oil, allow bacteria to grow and multiply in the follicle. This leads to inflammation. Enzymes from these bacteria themselves go on to cause more damage, which then leads to a breakdown of the hair follicle and an abscess forms.

Although you can use creams and medication, which can help to lessen the acne in the short term, the most effective long-term treatment involves tackling the underlying root cause, which again is insulin resistance. Weight loss, exercise, and a low-GI diet all help to reduce the insulin resistance. If you really don't want to wait to get rid of acne, check out Chapter 7 for medications that can help.

Hair in all the wrong places

A change in hair growth usually manifests as excessive hair growth on parts of the body that ought not to be hairy on a woman. (The term for this pattern of hair growth is *hirsutism*.) You may find that you develop hairiness on your face, chest, stomach, and back. Hirsutism affects 5 percent to 10 percent of all women and a much higher percentage of women with PCOS.

Because physical appearance has so much to do with how people relate to each other, hirsutism can be a distressing experience. At the very least, you may be chronically stressed by the amount of time and money you spend removing unwanted hair, in a seemingly never-ending battle.

The cause of excessive hair growth in areas where you don't want it is the excess production of male hormones, itself brought on by insulin resistance. The condition is likely to get worse the more weight you gain. Creams and cosmetic treatments are available that you can use to alleviate the problem, but to get rid of the underlying cause, you need to reduce insulin resistance by losing weight, which is best coupled with a low-GI diet and physical activity.

Unfortunately, in addition to gaining hair in places where you don't want it, with PCOS you're more likely to lose it on your head, a condition known as *alopecia*. Don't worry: You aren't going to go completely bald! What tends to happen with PCOS is that you get a gradual overall thinning of the hair, or thinning at the corners above the temple. As thinning continues the hair may go see-through so that it looks like a fine, fuzzy halo when light shines on it.

If you do suffer from alopecia, it's rarely severe and can be controlled by bringing down your male hormone levels by following the diet and exercise advice in this book (in the short term, your medical practitioner may also prescribe medication to do this).

Losing around 100 hairs a day is normal. Keep this in mind before you convince yourself you have alopecia just by looking at the few stray hairs in the sink.

Other potential symptoms

A number of less common symptoms also can effect you if you have PCOS, including the following:

✔ **Dizziness and fainting:** The dizziness and fainting associated with PCOS can be linked to the exhaustion that often occurs, but blood sugar levels that drop abnormally low also can cause dizziness and fainting. A low-GI diet helps to alleviate low blood sugars (see Chapter 4 for more about the ideal diet for PCOS).

✔ **Pain:** PCOS doesn't result in the type of pelvic pain that is sometimes associated with larger ovarian cysts, but you may notice some pelvic discomfort at times. This may be due to the effect of hormones on the flow of blood through the pelvic veins.

✔ **Migraines:** Hormonal issues often are related to migraines, so it's not surprising that women with PCOS often suffer from migraine headaches.

Psychological Symptoms

The psychological symptoms you get with PCOS can be as a result of having an illness that can have so many physical manifestations. Even the most naturally cheery of souls can feel down in the dumps from time to time. Some experts believe that the syndrome itself can have mind-altering effects — and not the pleasant "far out, man" type!

Emotional manifestations

If you have PCOS, you're more likely to suffer from depression, anxiety, irritability, and mood swings. In fact, it can seem as if you have premenstrual syndrome (PMS; characterized by a wide array of symptoms including irritability, anxiety, and wild fluctuations in mood); the difference is that in PCOS, the symptoms don't just appear before a period.

The emotional symptoms that accompany PCOS may be due to one, or all, of the following:

✔ Hormone disturbances

✔ A host of upsetting symptoms caused by PCOS

✔ The stress of living with a long-term medical condition

Another emotional manifestation of PCOS is the tendency toward eating disorders. A link exists between having an abnormal eating behavior and PCOS. Binge eating and bulimia are more common than in the general population — 1 percent of women have bulimia in the general population, whereas 6 percent of women who have

PCOS are bulimic. For detailed information about eating disorders and PCOS, head to Chapter 5.

Depression

One of the less recognized symptoms of PCOS is depression. Depression is more likely if you have more extreme symptoms of PCOS. Although depression stems from many factors, considering PCOS as a possible cause is always a good idea if you experience other PCOS symptoms as well.

Many experts are unclear as to whether depression really is a symptom of PCOS or whether your PCOS symptoms (such as weight gain and so on) cause depression. Whichever comes first — the depression or the PCOS — a vicious cycle can develop because the depression makes you less likely to want to deal with your PCOS symptoms, so they get worse, and as the symptoms get worse, so does the depression.

If you experience even some of the following symptoms of depression, seek help from your doctor:

✔ Feeling down, for no apparent reason, for more than a couple days in a row, especially if you feel far more down than any possible trigger warrants

✔ Avoiding having a social life, preferring to stay at home by yourself, and inventing excuses not to go out with friends or visit family

✔ Experiencing crying episodes, often for no real reason

✔ Having persistent trouble sleeping

✔ Being overly critical of yourself

✔ Having suicidal thoughts

Depression also can be a side effect of drugs that you may have been given to treat your PCOS. At least a hundred fairly common prescription drugs can bring about the side effect of depression. If you're feeling depressed, mention it to your doctor. If the cause is due to the drugs you're on, he may well be able to find alternative medications.

Some doctors prescribe antidepressants to treat depression in women with PCOS. These drugs don't alleviate the underlying issues, but they may help you to get motivated to tackle your PCOS.

Irritability, mood swings, and other psychological symptoms

In PCOS, the following symptoms sometimes appear on their own; sometimes they accompany PCOS-related depression (explained in the preceding section):

- ✔ Feeling stressed
- ✔ Feeling anxious
- ✔ Feeling out of control
- ✔ Experiencing a lack of mental alertness
- ✔ Experiencing a decreased sex drive

Binge eating and bulimia

Having PCOS seems to make you more prone to developing abnormal eating patterns. The most common effect is the desire to binge. In fact, up to 60 percent of women with bulimia have been found to have PCOS.

The binge-eating/bulimia cycle is a vicious one. You binge and then feel so guilty for bingeing that you do one of the following:

- ✔ Starve yourself until you can't hold out without food any longer.
- ✔ Try to get rid of the excess food you've eaten by making yourself sick.
- ✔ Try to get rid of the excess food you've eaten by taking lots of laxatives.

What normally happens after this is that you're either so hungry or so fed up that you binge all over again, and the cycle continues. Chapter 5 has more information on bingeing cycles. If you recognize a tendency in yourself to binge, you may need to seek some professional help in order to break out of this vicious cycle.

Detecting PCOS

PCOS is a tendency you're born with, so it can be lurking throughout your life, but you're statistically most likely to be diagnosed in your early- to mid-30s, perhaps because you're having difficulty conceiving.

Suspecting you have it

Because your doctor may not be looking for PCOS unless you go to her with complaints common to PCOS — such as infertility, absent periods, or acne — many women self-diagnose PCOS before they see their doctors. Self-diagnosis can be risky, though, if you diagnose a condition you don't actually have! If you think you have PCOS, talk with your gynecologist or your primary-care doctor before trying treatment that may not apply to your condition.

Even if your mother or sister has PCOS, and you think that you do, too, don't expect to have exactly the same symptoms. Symptoms of PCOS vary between women, even within the same family. So, your sister with PCOS may have periods, whereas you may have none at all. Also, your symptoms may change over time; expect them to get worse and expect more symptoms to develop if your weight continues to increase.

You can't really diagnose yourself with PCOS; if you think you have it, you need to get properly diagnosed by your doctor or specialist because other conditions have symptoms that are shared with PCOS. These other conditions include

- **PMS,** which occurs in many women from 2 to 14 days before the onset of menstruation and is characterized by a wide array of physical and mental symptoms.

- **Low thyroid function,** known as *hypothyroidism,* where the thyroid gland in the neck doesn't produce enough thyroid hormone. This condition can result in your feeling tired, perpetually cold, and putting on weight.

- **Adrenal deficiency,** also known as Addison's disease, which is a hormone deficiency caused by damage to the outer layer of the adrenal gland and results in your feeling weak and tired.

- **Cushing's syndrome,** caused by increased production of cortisol, or by excessive use of cortisol or other steroid hormones. Weakness, acne, and weight gain are common symptoms.

- **Hyperprolactinemia,** characterized by increased levels of the hormone prolactin in the blood. Women with this condition mainly experience disrupted or absent periods and infertility.

- **Androgen-producing tumors,** which result in the production of high levels of male hormone, particularly testosterone.

Getting a doctor's clarification

If you suspect that you have PCOS, your doctor or gynecologist can help you determine a diagnosis. In addition to taking a medical history from you and conducting a physical examination, she may look for at least two symptoms of PCOS. According to the American Society for Reproductive Medicine, PCOS is defined by the presence of any two of the following characteristics:

- Lack of ovulation for an extended period of time (which probably manifests itself as the stopping of your monthly period)
- High levels of androgens
- Many small cysts on the ovaries

Your own doctor may need to send you for some tests in order to detect if any of these are occurring. These tests may include a number of the different procedures covered in the following sections.

Scan of the ovaries

A woman's ovaries are where her eggs are stored. Each egg is stored in a capsule called a follicle. Once a month, many follicles begin to grow. Only one matures to produce an egg, which is released at ovulation. In normal circumstances, the follicles that didn't fully mature that month dissolve. In PCOS, none of the eggs mature fully; they remain at a size of about 2 to 9 millimeters in diameter within a fluid-filled cyst. (A mature follicle that is ready to release an egg reaches 20+ millimeters in diameter.)

Over time, the ovaries fill with many cysts, and this is why PCOS is described as *polycystic,* which means "many cysts." These small cysts in the ovaries don't get larger; in fact, they eventually disappear and are replaced by new cysts.

In order to look at the ovaries, an ultrasound scan is done. This procedure uses safe, high-frequency sound waves and allows an image of the ovaries to be seen on a special computer. The ultrasound can detect if a woman's ovaries are enlarged (which can happen in PCOS) or if cysts are present. This sort of scan also can pick up a thickening of the endometrium.

Hormone tests

Your medical practitioner or specialist may suggest you have some blood work done. These tests show any disturbed levels of the hormones controlling ovulation and give an indication that PCOS may be the problem.

Hormones are substances that get released into your bloodstream and circulate around the body, influencing other organs. In PCOS, the hormones that control ovulation are out of balance, such as progesterone (too little is produced), androgens (too much is produced), and luteinizing hormone (too much is produced).

Luteinizing hormone (LH) is an important hormone throughout the cycle because it influences hormone production and acts as a trigger for ovulation. The disrupted hormone levels cause period irregularities. Another hormone called *follicle stimulating hormone* (FSH) should be in the right proportion to LH. Doctors can measure the ratio of LH to FSH and use it as a means of monitoring the condition and whether various treatment options are working. See Chapter 10 for more on the inner workings of hormones that govern the menstrual cycle and affect your ability to get pregnant.

The glucose tolerance test explained

If you have diabetes, or even severe insulin resistance, the body is unable to make normal use of glucose as fuel, and it accumulates in high amounts in the blood. Even in healthy people, glucose levels in the blood rise after a meal, but they soon return to normal as the glucose is used up or stored. A glucose tolerance test (GTT) can distinguish between the normal pattern of clearing glucose and what happens if diabetes or severe insulin resistance (sometimes known as glucose intolerance or prediabetes) is present.

A GTT is performed after an overnight fast. The GTT can be done in several ways, but typically, a sample of your blood is taken, and your blood glucose level is measured. Then you're asked to drink a standard amount of glucose, usually 75 grams, dissolved in water. Two hours later, you have another blood sample taken and the blood glucose level is measured again. The levels of glucose in the two samples are then carefully measured.

A diagnosis of diabetes is made if the level of glucose is over a set level:

✔ If the fasting blood sample is over 126 mg/dL

✔ If the level of the sample taken two hours after a 75-gram glucose drink is more than 140 mg/dL

Approximately 20 percent to 40 percent of women with PCOS have an abnormal glucose tolerance test.

During pregnancy, many women also have a glucose tolerance test done. If a screening test called a glucose challenge test comes back abnormally high, a three-hour GTT is done, using a 100-gram dose of glucose. Gestational diabetes increases your chance of later developing type 2 diabetes and also increases the risk of having a child who will later be overweight — which can, in turn, increase your child's chances of having PCOS, if you have a daughter who is susceptible to the disorder.

The tests go on and on . . .

Your doctor may check certain other blood levels, which are often out of kilter in PCOS. These tests may include the following:

- ✔ **Glucose tolerance test:** Checks whether you can cope with a certain load of sugar. If your body is not coping very well with a sugar load, this is an indication that you have, or are on the threshold of developing, type 2 diabetes. (See the nearby sidebar for more on this test.)

- ✔ **Fasting glucose level:** If your body has not been able to bring down glucose levels to a normal value first thing in the morning before eating, this can also be a sign that you have diabetes or are borderline.

- ✔ **Insulin testing:** It's possible to test your insulin levels for abnormalities as well. If you have insulin resistance, normally your fasting insulin level is elevated.

- ✔ **Blood cholesterol measurements:** These can include measurements of cholesterol and bad fats (called *triglycerides*) that circulate in the blood.

PCOS through Life's Changes

Your PCOS symptoms will probably change with each stage of your life. Symptoms will get worse if you gain extra weight and may get worse if you get stressed or ill. But are you stuck with PCOS for life?

Well, yes and no. No cure exists for PCOS, and if you make no changes to your lifestyle, you could well have to deal with symptoms throughout your entire life. But you can rid yourself of symptoms by changing your lifestyle into a healthy one, whether you're 14 or 40!

The first warning signs: Puberty

PCOS doesn't just suddenly appear; it's a disorder that is present throughout life. However, it may not manifest itself until puberty, when you first start having menstrual periods or, rather, *should* start having menstrual periods.

Diagnosing PCOS in young teenage girls is not a clear-cut thing, because during puberty the hormones are jumping all over the place anyway and the body goes through some fairly major changes. Weight gain, acne, and irregular periods are all common female teenage traits.

Going through adolescence is tough enough with all the normal hormonal changes that go on, but it can be harder still when this time heralds the start of PCOS symptoms. If the tendency to develop PCOS exists, weight gain during this time may act as a trigger to developing the condition.

If PCOS runs in the family, keep an eye out for any developing symptoms. Watch particularly for rapid weight gain and periods that start and then stop for months on end, or that occur at very irregular intervals.

Weight gain needs to be tackled sensitively — all teens need to avoid it, but particularly so if it's likely to set off the full-blown syndrome. However, teenagers hate being lectured to, and you need to be careful to avoid triggering abnormal eating patterns and eating disorders. Talk to your daughter in terms of her health, not in terms of her appearance.

Pregnancy and PCOS

Unfortunately, PCOS can put you at increased risk of having a miscarriage, of developing gestational diabetes, and also of developing *pregnancy toxemia* (also known as pre-eclampsia, where blood pressure can reach a dangerously high level for both mother and baby). Gestational diabetes is a transient diabetes that occurs in pregnant women, particularly if they're overweight at the start of pregnancy and/or gain a lot of weight during pregnancy. Women who have gestational diabetes have an increased risk of developing type 2 diabetes in the future.

Being in the best possible shape prior to getting pregnant helps prevent any pregnancy problems and may help to reduce the risk of miscarriage. (Chapter 11 talks about some of the complications of pregnancy when you have PCOS.) Getting down to your target weight prior to pregnancy and avoiding excessive weight gain during pregnancy can help to offset the risk of developing gestational diabetes.

Menopause and beyond

Menopause is the time when you have your last period and fertility ends. The average age of menopause in the developed world is 51. However, the wind down to menopause can happen for a number of years before periods actually end for good, and this time period is known as *peri-menopause*. Peri-menopause is characterized by often irregular periods and fluctuating hormone levels.

The danger of weight gain during adolescence

Recent research shows that, during the transition to puberty, weight gain that leads to obesity is associated with an increased production of androgens — a possible forerunner to the development of PCOS and a sign that insulin resistance is occurring.

In the girls measured who had gained weight and become obese, total testosterone levels (testosterone is the dominant male hormone) were over twice as high as those in normal-weight girls. Obesity in childhood is associated with insulin resistance, raised blood pressure, and adverse changes in blood fat levels, which may lead to future heart health problems.

However, doctors are now realizing that obesity may also be predisposing these girls to PCOS along with all its problems, including cosmetic problems such as hairiness, delayed or irregular periods, and later problems of infertility. The increase in overweight and obesity and teens in America today could trigger an explosion in the number of cases of PCOS in the next few years.

You may find it difficult to distinguish peri-menopause symptoms from PCOS symptoms because they include

- A tendency to gain weight
- Irregular periods, which can get heavier or lighter
- Hot flashes
- Fluctuating hormone levels, which can bring about mood changes

Unfortunately, hitting menopause doesn't mean that PCOS suddenly goes away. What tends to happen is that symptoms remain that predispose you to developing heart disease. These symptoms include weight gain around the middle, insulin resistance, type 2 diabetes, metabolic syndrome, and distorted blood fat levels (a condition known as *dislipidemia*).

Women with PCOS are more likely to be at risk for cardiovascular disorders, including atherosclerosis, heart attack and high blood pressure after menopause from these conditions. Complications from type 2 diabetes also continue to progress after menopause, since most diabetic complications worsen over time.

Because weight tends to increase after menopause even in women without PCOS, postmenopausal women with PCOS need to be extra vigilant to keep weight under control. Continue to follow the low-GI diet after menopause to keep both your weight and your blood glucose levels within normal limits.

Evidence exists that the high androgen levels remain after menopause, so male-pattern hair growth on the face and other parts of the body also remain. Because women often develop extra hair growth on their face after menopause, having PCOS just worsens this common postmenopausal side effect.

Part II
Taking Control of Your Symptoms

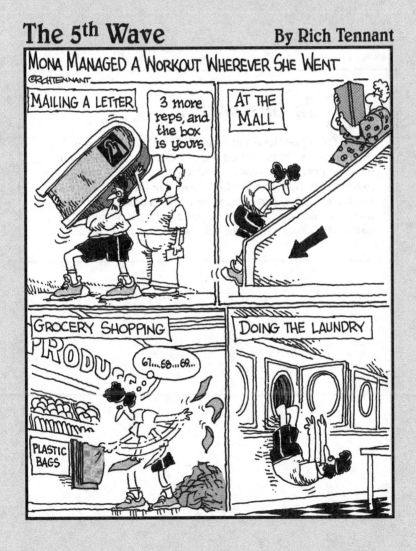

The 5th Wave   By Rich Tennant

MONA MANAGED A WORKOUT WHEREVER SHE WENT

MAILING A LETTER — 3 more reps, and the box is yours.

AT THE MALL

GROCERY SHOPPING — 67...68...69...

PLASTIC BAGS

DOING THE LAUNDRY

In this part...

When you have a chronic disease that affects as many areas of your life as PCOS does, finding out what you can do to control and improve your symptoms is essential. In this part, we talk about the incredible benefits of diet, exercise, and keeping your mind and body in balance. We also review the different medications and alternative treatments that can help when you have PCOS.

Chapter 3

Coping with Insulin Resistance and Its Effects

*I*nsulin plays an essential part in the uptake of glucose into cells where it can be used for energy. Insulin is such an essential hormone that lack of it can lead to *hyperglycemia* (high glucose levels) and death. When cells develop insulin resistance, they no longer respond to the release of insulin by taking up glucose. This leads to high glucose levels, which, in turn, leads to a multitude of undesirable health effects.

In this chapter, we explain how insulin resistance develops, its health effects, and, most important, how you can combat it.

Defining Insulin Resistance

Insulin resistance is a complex condition that causes most of the symptoms of PCOS. Insulin resistance is not rare — it affects around 3 percent of people. In the normal metabolic process, the pancreas releases insulin in response to ingestion of food and the appearance of glucose in the bloodstream. In insulin resistance, this process, for a number of reasons, goes awry.

How insulin works

Insulin is a hormone produced by the pancreas, an organ that produces hormones and digestive enzymes. High levels of glucose in the blood stimulate the release of insulin from the pancreas.

An average balanced meal proves around 90 grams of carbohydrate, released over a period of around two hours. Insulin released in response to glucose facilitates uptake of glucose into cells and also helps convert excess glucose into glycogen. Glycogen is stored in the liver; some excess glucose is also converted to fat.

Abnormal insulin patterns

Abnormal insulin release patterns fall into two types:

- ✔ **Too little or no insulin production:** In type 1 diabetes, insulin-producing cells are destroyed by antibodies as part of an autoimmune response. In type 2 diabetes, insulin-producing cells "burn out" over time and not enough insulin is produced. In both cases, glucose levels in the blood rise.

- ✔ **Too much insulin production, or** *hyperinsulinemia:* Overproduction of insulin occurs when cells become resistant to the effects of insulin. The pancreas tried to "force" the cells to take up glucose by putting out more insulin. Over time, the overproduction of insulin wears out the insulin-producing cells, and insulin production drops.

Why insulin resistance develops

The question of why insulin resistance develops in the first place is complex, but the following are factors that contribute to development of insulin resistance:

- ✔ **Genetics:** Certain genes may contribute to insulin resistance and type 2 diabetes.

- ✔ **Being overweight:** Weight that accumulates around the waist, in particular, is associated with insulin resistance.

- ✔ **Abnormal lipids:** High levels of triglycerides and cholesterol in the blood also increase the chance of developing insulin resistance.

- ✔ **High blood pressure:** Medically known as *hypertension,* high blood pressure contributes to the development of insulin resistance.

- ✔ **High levels of cortisol in the blood:** Stress and high levels of meat intake are two causes of high cortisol levels. Cortisol counteracts insulin, which contributes to insulin resistance.

Diagnosing Insulin Resistance

Insulin resistance is an important indicator for the risk of developing type 2 diabetes. By the time blood sugar levels rise and diabetes is diagnosed, a number of cells that produce insulin in the pancreas may already have been destroyed. Diagnosing insulin resistance early and treating it before cells that produce insulin are irrevocably damaged may delay or prevent the onset of type 2 diabetes.

Insulin blood test results

Simple fasting insulin levels can be used to show the presence of insulin resistance with reasonable accuracy. Lab values vary, but many practitioners follow these guidelines for fasting insulin levels:

- ✔ **Normal:** Less than 10 mIU/mL

- ✔ **Some insulin resistance:** Between 10 mIU/mL and 14 mIU/mL

- ✔ **Insulin resistance:** Greater than 15 mIU/mL

 Diagnosing insulin resistance sometimes require a complex blood test involving simultaneous infusion of insulin and glucose called a *hyperinsulinemic euglycemic clamp study,* but this is rarely necessary outside of laboratory studies.

Physical signs

There aren't a lot of physical signs of insulin resistance, but the following clues can warn you of the possibility:

- ✔ **Development of *acanthosis nigricans* (darkened areas of skin around the neck, in the armpits, on the elbows, behind the knees, and around the knuckles):** Although acanthosis nigricans can have other causes, insulin resistance is a common cause.

- ✔ **Fat accumulation around the waist, called *central obesity.***

- ✔ **Skin tags that grow off the skin.**

Other symptoms of insulin resistance that may affect some people and not others include the following:

- ✔ Brain fogginess or difficulty concentrating

- ✔ Bloating and gas

- ✔ Depression

✔ Elevated triglyceride levels

✔ High blood pressure

✔ Increased appetite

✔ Weight gain

Diabetes and Insulin Resistance

The main concern with insulin resistance is the potential development of type 2 diabetes. Eating right, losing weight, and exercising are the keys to keep insulin resistance from developing into diabetes.

If you think making dietary and lifestyle changes can't help, chew on these facts:

✔ Just eating fewer calories lowers insulin resistance in days, even before you lose any weight.

✔ Losing 10 to 20 pounds has a substantial impact on blood glucose levels.

✔ Losing 16 percent of your body weight increases glucose metabolism by 100 percent.

✔ Exercise can increase insulin sensitivity for up to 16 hours afterward, according to at least one study.

Prediabetes: How diabetes sneaks up on you

Prediabetes, once called impaired glucose tolerance or impaired fasting glucose, the stage where your fasting blood glucose levels rise above normal but not high enough to be classified as diabetes, is common in insulin resistance.

Prediabetes is diagnosed in two different ways:

✔ **Fasting blood sugar:** If you have fasting blood glucose levels between 100 mg/dL and 125 mg/dL, you have prediabetes.

✔ **Glucose tolerance test (GTT):** In a GTT, a fasting blood glucose level is drawn, followed by ingestion of 75 grams of glucose in a drink or snack. Blood is drawn again after two hours. A blood glucose level between 140 mg/dL and 199 mg/dL two hours after drinking the high-glucose drink is diagnostic for prediabetes.

Prediabetes requires special vigilance. It's easy to not pay much attention or take any action when your blood glucose is "only" 101 or 102 mg/dL compared to the norm of less than 100 mg/dL, but this is the stage where your efforts can slow or prevent the onset of type 2 diabetes.

Once you develop prediabetes, chances are, you'll develop type 2 diabetes within the next ten years unless you lose between 5 percent and 7 percent of your body weight.

Nearly everyone who develops type 2 diabetes has prediabetes first. But prediabetes doesn't have to develop into diabetes. According to the American Diabetes Association, exercising for 30 minutes a day combined with weight loss of 5 percent to 10 percent of body weight reduces the risk of developing diabetes by 58 percent.

If you have prediabetes, don't wait for your blood sugars to get worse before taking action. Start following the low-GI diet outlined in Chapter 4 and implement the weight-loss tips in Chapter 5 to ward off diabetes for as long as possible — and possibly forever.

Insulin burnout

Over time, the constant stimulation of the beta cells in the pancreas to produce insulin wears out the cells. Eventually, they burn out and can no longer produce enough insulin to remove glucose from the bloodstream. When this happens, blood glucose levels rise to levels high enough to be classified as diabetes. Burned-out insulin cells can't repair themselves, so diabetes doesn't go away once it develops, although you can modify its effects with weight loss, diet, and exercise.

Because type 2 diabetes is a lifelong condition that can't be reversed, only controlled, preventing it from developing is the best defense against a lifetime of potential complications from diabetes.

Developing Type 2 Diabetes

Type 2 diabetes is far and away the most common type of diabetes in the United States. Over 90 percent of diabetes is type 2 diabetes. Unlike type 1 diabetes, which occurs as a result of an autoimmune disorder, the risks for type 2 diabetes can be modified. Around 8.3 percent of the U.S. adult population had diabetes in 2011; as many as seven million people with diabetes have not been diagnosed and don't know they have it.

Identifying the main causes of type 2 diabetes

Many factors contribute to diabetes. The top risk factors include the following:

- ✔ **Obesity:** Ninety percent of people with diabetes are at least 20 percent overweight

- ✔ **Family history of type 2 diabetes in a parent or sibling**

- ✔ **History of impaired glucose tolerance**

- ✔ **History of PCOS**

- ✔ **Being of Hispanic, Native American, African American, Asian American, or Pacific Islander descent**

- ✔ **Being over age 45,** although type 2 diabetes is being diagnosed at younger and younger ages

Realizing you have type 2 diabetes

Symptoms of diabetes can be subtle and easily missed, which is why at least 6 million people with diabetes, or around 33 percent of those who have the disease, are undiagnosed and untreated. Symptoms you may notice include the following:

- ✔ **Increased thirst:** The high sugar levels in your blood pulls fluid from your tissues to dilute it, so you feel thirsty.

- ✔ **Increased urination:** As you drink more, you urinate more.

- ✔ **Weight loss:** Even though you have high levels of glucose in your blood, it can't get into the cells because you no longer produce enough insulin to effectively transport glucose into cells. Your body breaks down fat for energy instead, so you lose weight.

- ✔ **Blurred vision:** Because fluid is pulled from the lenses of your eye, you may not be able to focus well, and your vision becomes blurry.

- ✔ **Fatigue:** Diabetes causes fatigue because your cells aren't getting the energy they need in the form of glucose.

- ✔ **Increased risk of infection or slow-healing sores:** High amounts of sugar in the blood interfere with healing.

- ✔ **Increased appetite:** Despite the high glucose levels in the blood, your cells are starving, so you feel hungry.

Eating right to control blood sugars

Changing your diet is an essential part of treating diabetes. Diabetics need glucose, but they need the right types of glucose, which is where the low glycemic index diet comes in. (See Chapter 4 for the rundown on how to eat the low-GI way.) You also need to watch your glucose intake once you develop type 2 diabetes. If you want to avoid taking medication to control your blood sugar levels, diet and exercise are your best bets.

At one time, the American Diabetes Association advocated a diet system that counted carbohydrates, assigning points to different carbs. Today, the emphasis is more on individually planned diets. When planning a diabetic diet, consider the follow guidelines, according to the American Diabetic Association:

✔ Fill half your plate with non-starchy vegetables and then add protein to fill 25 percent of the plate and whole grains to fill the other 25 percent.

✔ Add a side of fruit and a serving of low-fat dairy to your meal-time intake.

✔ Avoid refined carbohydrates, which are low in nutrients and high in calories.

✔ Keep your fat intake to 30 percent of your daily calorie intake, and restrict your saturated fat intake.

You may notice something about today's diabetic diet — it's pretty similar to the recommendations we make for a healthy PCOS diet as well! Choose foods with a low glycemic index to help stabilize your blood sugar levels and you'll be eating a healthy diabetic diet without having to count carbohydrates.

Avoiding the long-term effects of diabetes

The long-term effects of diabetes can be severe. Although it may take ten years or more for the complications of diabetes to manifest themselves, when your blood glucose levels are out of control, the damage is done day by day, little by little, over time.

Diabetics normally can't keep their fasting and *post-prandial* (after eating) blood glucose levels as low as people without diabetes can, but keeping your levels within the range set by your doctor, who knows your case best, can help avoid the serious and even life-threatening complications of diabetes.

Diabetes affects blood vessels in a number of ways. Both small and large blood vessels are affected. *Microvascular effects* (which affect the small blood vessels) include problems with the kidneys, the nervous system, and the small vessels in the eye. *Macrovascular effects* (which affect the large blood vessels) include heart disease such as atherosclerosis, coronary artery disease, and stroke. The following sections detail the potential specific effects of diabetes.

Cardiovascular complications

Diabetics have double the risk of developing heart problems over people who don't have diabetes. Blood vessels are damaged by high levels of circulating glucose, which makes them more prone to *atherosclerosis*, the buildup of plaque inside the blood vessels that narrows the arteries and restricts blood flow to the heart. Blood clots can develop at the sites of atherosclerosis; clots can break loose and block blood flow to the heart or brain, causing heart attack or stroke.

The heart muscle itself can become damaged over time from high levels of glucose. Reduced blood flow to the heart because of atherosclerosis also can cause heart failure. People with diabetes have double the risk of heart failure compared to people without diabetes.

High blood pressure is also common in diabetics because of narrowing of the blood vessels and damage to the heart or the blood vessel walls.

Diabetic retinopathy

Around 10,000 diabetics in the United States go blind each year from the effects of diabetic retinopathy, according to the American Diabetes Association. *Retinopathy,* or damage to the blood vessels in the *retina* (the part of the eye that contains the sensors that transmit signals through the optic nerve to your brain), can start as early as seven years before a person is diagnosed with type 2 diabetes.

Common vision problems in diabetics include swelling and bleeding into parts of the retina, which interferes with vision. The retina can become detached from the back of the eye if new abnormal blood vessels form and pull the retina away from the wall. Bleeding into the *vitreous* (the fluid in the middle of the eye that helps shape the eye) can block light from entering the eye. When light can't enter, you can't see.

Kidney disease

Diabetes accounts for almost 44 percent of all new cases of kidney failure and is the most common disease related to kidney failure. Normally, kidney failure takes 15 to 25 years to develop in diabetes. Kidney disease occurs when high levels of glucose damage the cells within the kidney. *Hypertension,* common in diabetics, also contributes to kidney disease. In a catch-22, kidney disease also worsens hypertension.

Keeping both blood sugar levels and blood pressure low can help prevent kidney damage and avoid the need for dialysis or kidney transplant.

Diabetic neuropathy

Damage to the small blood vessels often has the greatest effect on the small blood vessels in the extremities — the hands, feet, arms, and legs. At least 60 percent of all diabetics develop some type of neuropathy, which is most common in people who have had diabetes for at least 25 years.

Peripheral neuropathy can cause loss of sensation in the extremities. In the feet, a lack of feeling can lead to small injuries and breaks in the skin being ignored until infection sets in. Because diabetics also have less ability to fight off infection due to high glucose levels in the blood, serious infections can lead to amputation of feet and even part of the legs if not treated promptly.

Nerve damage can affect all the major organs and can lead to muscle loss, constipation, urinary problems, pain, weakness, or loss of balance and coordination.

Putting the genie back in the bottle: Controlling diabetes

Once type 2 diabetes develops, can you ever get rid of it or at least control it to the point where you don't need medication? Yes, definitely, as long as you still produce insulin on your own and don't require insulin injections. Reversing the effects of diabetes requires controlling your blood sugars, and you already know the answer to how to do that — it takes a combination of the right diet and exercise to achieve good glycemic control.

Will you always have to watch what you eat, how much you weigh and commit to an exercise program for the rest of your life? Yes, probably. But considering the complications that can develop when your blood sugars are allowed to rage out of control for a few years, the effort will be worth it.

Metabolic Syndrome: Insulin Resistance Plus a Whole Lot More

Metabolic syndrome is a fairly new name for what is also called insulin resistance syndrome or syndrome X. Metabolic syndrome is a constellation of symptoms that can develop when insulin resistance affects different organs and body systems. In many ways, the effects of metabolic syndrome and type 2 diabetes are similar.

Assessing different criteria

One problem with metabolic syndrome is that there's no agreement on exactly which symptoms should be considered for inclusion when diagnosing the disorder. The World Health Organization, the American Heart Association, the U.S. National Cholesterol Education Program Adult Treatment Panel, and the International Diabetes Federation all have their own ideas about what to include, but they all agree on certain central points, including the ones covered in this section.

The American Heart Association and the National Heart, Lung, and Blood Institute agree that you need to have three or more of the following symptoms for diagnosis.

Central obesity

Central obesity, or increased waist circumference is included in every definition, although groups define it differently. For women, an increased waist circumference is anywhere from approximately 31½ inches for the European Group for the Study of Insulin Resistance to 35 inches for the American Heart Association or the National Cholesterol Education Program Adult Treatment Panel.

The International Diabetes Foundations goes one step further and says that if you have a body mass index (BMI) greater than 30, central obesity is assumed and waist measurements are not necessary.

You can go to www.nhlbisupport.com/bmi to calculate your BMI.

Elevated lipids

Lipids, which include cholesterol and triglycerides, are also an integral part of diagnosis for all the groups that define metabolic syndrome. Most define an elevated triglyceride level as 150 mg/dL or above. High-density lipoprotein (HDL), the "good" cholesterol, of below 50 mg/dL for women is also considered to be part of metabolic syndrome.

Identifying a new disorder

Defining the existence of metabolic syndrome was a group effort stretching over a number of years. Different doctors over the years identified different pieces of metabolic syndrome, which was first termed "metabolic syndrome" by Hermann Haller in 1977. In 1988, Gerald Reaven first associated the disorder with insulin resistance and termed it "syndrome X."

Unfortunately, the knowledge of the causes and a specific name for the disorder didn't solve the problem of exactly which criteria constitute the disease; the World Health Organization, the International Diabetes Federation, and the American Heart Association, among others, all have their own inclusion criteria for diagnosis of metabolic disorder, while some critics claim that, although certain symptoms are generally found together, they don't constitute a new disease.

High blood pressure

High blood pressure, or hypertension, is considered part of the diagnostic criteria for metabolic syndrome by every group, although some set the limits at 130/85 mmHg and others at 140/90 mmHg.

Fasting glucose levels

Fasting blood glucose levels are another point of agreement by all the groups with diagnostic criteria for metabolic syndrome. Levels over 100 mg/dL or previous diagnosis of type 2 diabetes are considered to be evidence of the disorder when seen with other criteria. As many as 75 percent of people with abnormal glucose levels may have metabolic syndrome.

Other factors

The World Health Organization adds protein in the urine or an elevated albumin-to-creatinine ratio, both signs of kidney damage, as a potential indicator of metabolic syndrome. Fatty liver (which can be seen on ultrasound and which affects as many as 66 percent of all obese American adults), high uric acid levels in the blood, and the presence of polycystic ovaries are often associated with metabolic syndrome as well. Blood tests may show elevated levels of C-reactive protein, associated with inflammation in the blood vessels.

Pondering potential heart problems

Metabolic syndrome obviously increases the risk of diabetes, because elevated blood sugars are one of the main criteria for diagnosis, but metabolic syndrome also can have serious effects on your heart.

As many as 50 percent of people with coronary heart disease, which affects the blood vessels leading to the heart, have metabolic syndrome. Metabolic syndrome can increase your risk of heart disease in several ways.

Heart attack

People with metabolic syndrome are three times as likely to have a heart attack and are twice as likely to die from a heart attack as those without the syndrome. Coronary artery disease causes 1.5 million heart attacks each year; 33 percent are fatal.

High blood pressure

High blood pressure is one of the symptoms of metabolic syndrome. When blood pressure is high, the heart has to pump harder to move blood through the vessels to the tissues. Pushing blood with more force damages the blood vessel walls, which makes them more susceptible to developing atherosclerosis. Pumping with extra force also tires the heart muscle, which may first grow larger in an effort to pump harder. Over time, the heart muscle may become weak from working so hard.

Weak heart muscle

When the heart muscle weakens, each pump of the heart forces a reduced amount of blood through the ventricles. Blood begins to back up in the heart and lungs, causing edema and swelling of the extremities (called *right-sided failure*) or fluid in the lungs (called *left-sided failure*).

Atherosclerosis

As insulin comes in contact with the interior wall of your arteries, it can damage the walls, causing the initial injury that produces plaque that builds up in the arteries. Plaque formation leads to atherosclerosis. If the arteries leading to your heart get blocked due to the plaque formation, it results in a heart attack. If the plaque builds up in the arteries leading to your brain, or if clots that form at the site break off and travel to the brain, it results in a stroke.

Abnormal cholesterol levels, high levels of C-reactive protein, and a tendency toward increased blood clotting all increase the risk of developing atherosclerosis.

Focusing on fatty liver

The metabolic syndrome group of disorders also appears to increase the risk of developing nonalcoholic fatty liver disease (NAFLD). NAFLD affects as many as 66 percent of people diagnosed as obese and may affect even more people who have metabolic syndrome.

NAFLD can progress to nonalcoholic steatohepatitis (NASH), a more serious disease that can lead to fibrosis, scarring in the liver, and eventually cirrhosis and liver failure.

Fatty liver also increases the risk of both heart disease and type 2 diabetes because a fatty liver increases levels of very low density lipoprotein (VLDL), glucose, C-reactive protein, and factors that increase blood clotting.

Chapter 4

The Glycemic Index and Diet

In This Chapter

▶ Eating the low-GI way

▶ Planning low-GI meals

▶ Understanding that it doesn't just end at low-GI eating

*D*iet can have a big impact on PCOS. Although good nutrition can benefit everyone, it's especially important when you have insulin resistance (see Chapter 3 for a complete discussion of what insulin resistance means). Because many women with PCOS do have insulin resistance, concentrating on foods that have a low glycemic index (GI) can improve insulin resistance. A low-GI diet also may help you knock off some pounds, which can improve your symptoms.

In this chapter, I explain what the glycemic index is and why keeping certain types of carbohydrates under control in your diet will benefit you. But following a certain type of diet is only part of the story when talking about nutrition and PCOS. I also delve into the importance of fats and other nutrients in your diet and tell you how to choose wisely. Diet is a weighty subject, but one you'll be glad you tackled.

The Basics about Low-GI Diets

A low-GI diet is one where the carbohydrates you consume break down slowly and/or slowly release glucose into your bloodstream so that your blood glucose levels remain stable. Evidence suggests that a low-GI diet also may help you to eat less because you feel less hungry between or before meals. Because both insulin resistance and diabetes often are part of PCOS, all are helped by keeping blood glucose levels stable. PCOS sufferers also have a tendency to feel quite hungry and gain weight easily, so a low-GI diet is ideal for curtailing this problem.

The GI concept is a fairly recent one that started in the early 1970s when scientists began to look at how different carbohydrates affect the blood glucose in different ways. Then, in 1981, a Canadian doctor, David Jenkins, and his team expanded this work; they saw that some carbs send blood glucose levels shooting up wildly almost straight after consumption, whereas other carbs cause hardly a blip in blood glucose levels. The research into the effect that fast or slow blood glucose rises have on humans who are healthy, as well as on humans who have impaired blood glucose controls, still continues.

The low-GI diet is not just another dieting fad; it's backed by science. In this section, you find out how it can be the sensible way to eat for life — and not just if you have PCOS.

Research on the glycemic index

More and more research is coming out to support the following of a low-GI diet. It seems that the low-GI way to eat is great not just for those with PCOS, but also for the general population. This is particularly the case because more people are carrying around too much weight, developing high blood pressure, generating high cholesterol levels, and suffering other health problems. Following is a list of what some recent research has shown with regard to the general health gains achieved by following a low-GI diet:

- **Low-GI diets help people lose and control weight.** Research has shown that moderate reductions in GI make losing weight easier, particularly for women. This may be because low-GI foods may help keep away hunger pangs for longer due to their "slow-release" characteristic.

- **Low-GI diets increase the body's sensitivity to insulin.**

- **Low-GI carbs improve diabetes control.**

- **Low-GI carbs may be able to reduce the risk of heart disease.** Research shows that a high-carb diet based around low-GI foods is overall the most effective for heart health. Research also shows that low-GI whole-grain foods such as oatmeal provide heart health benefits over and above those of high-GI whole grains such as whole-wheat flakes.

- **Low-GI carbs reduce blood cholesterol levels and other harmful blood fats without lowering the body's good fat level — high-density lipoprotein (HDL).**

- **Low-GI diets may help to reduce the risk of getting certain cancers such as colorectal and breast cancer.**

- **Low-GI carbs can help prolong physical endurance (which is why sportsmen and women eat a low-GI diet before an event).**

Digest this!

As soon as you eat a food containing some carbohydrate, digestive enzymes in the saliva in your mouth start to break down the carbs in your food into simpler sugars. Starch, for example, is made up of long chains of glucose molecules. So, when starch is broken down, starting in the mouth, you get a release of free glucose. The breakdown process continues throughout the rest of the gut, with digestive enzymes getting released along the way, which gradually fully break down the more complicated food compounds. The chewing process in the mouth and churning process in the stomach (along with the mixing with stomach acid) also aid this breakdown of food.

Although the glycemic index concept is an important one if you have PCOS, it's not the be all and end all of diet tips and tricks. The GI should be incorporated into healthy eating guidelines, which we review throughout this chapter.

Identifying how GI affects your blood sugar

Different types of carbs affect your blood glucose level in different ways. Quick nutrition lesson: Food is broken down in your gut into smaller elements, and these elements are absorbed into the bloodstream. (Lucky for you, you only need to know how your body digests carbs, because only foods containing carbs — which includes sugars — affect your eventual blood glucose level.)

Your body can absorb carbs only when they are broken down into

- ✔ Glucose
- ✔ Fructose (found in high levels in fruit)
- ✔ Galactose (derived from milk)

Even relatively simple sugar products such as *sucrose* (table sugar) are broken down by the body to glucose and fructose.

The rate of breakdown and release of glucose into the bloodstream has the most influence on the GI of a food.

Seeing how GI affects PCOS

The graphs shown in Figure 4-1 demonstrate what happens in your bloodstream when you consume a food or drink with a high GI compared to one with a low GI. You can see that the glucose drink in the first graph, with a high GI of 100, requires so little breaking down by the body that the sugar it contains gets rapidly absorbed, almost all at once, and rushes quickly into the bloodstream, causing a rapid and sudden rise in blood glucose levels. The second graph shows blood glucose levels after eating spaghetti, with a GI of 41.

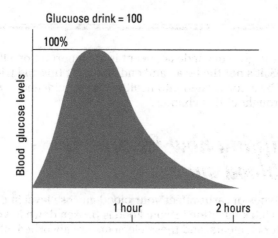

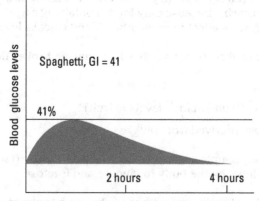

Figure 4-1: Comparing blood glucose levels after consuming a high-GI food and a low-GI food.

A sudden rise in blood sugar isn't terribly good news even when you don't have PCOS, but if you do have PCOS, the harmful effect gets exaggerated:

- ✔ **Your blood glucose level may stay elevated for extended periods of time.** When you suffer from PCOS, the body finds it difficult to bring down a high level of blood glucose, so it stays high for a long period of time, particularly if you have full-blown diabetes or insulin resistance. With diabetes, your body is unable to produce enough insulin to bring down the high glucose level, whereas in insulin resistance, insulin is produced but is unable to do its job of bringing down blood glucose levels very effectively. Over time, having high blood glucose levels can give rise to several complications, including heart disease, kidney failure, and damage to the eyes.

- ✔ **Your blood sugar may drop to a level where you start to notice yourself getting a little dysfunctional.** In some cases, when your body can still pump out insulin effectively, the body responds to high blood glucose levels by pumping out too much insulin. PCOS sufferers seem particularly susceptible to this happening. So, in some PCOS sufferers, a food that causes blood glucose to rise suddenly can cause a rebound effect where a high blood glucose level is followed by blood glucose levels plummeting too low. This sudden drop, called *hypoglycemia,* leads to feelings of shakiness, severe hunger, anxiety, and even fainting.

- ✔ **Your body overproduces insulin.** Most of the symptoms of PCOS are due to excessive levels of insulin being produced. This is because insulin is just not effective at normal levels due to a condition known as *insulin resistance.* Easing the symptoms of PCOS revolves around trying to reduce these excessive insulin levels. High-GI foods promote excess insulin secretion, which may increase the risk for diabetes, cardiovascular disease, and some types of cancer, as well as generally making the symptoms of PCOS worse.

- ✔ **You may become hungrier faster.** When the glucose from a meal is dumped all at once into your bloodstream, you're filled up for a while, but there's nothing sustainable about it; after your glucose levels return to normal (or even lower than normal), you may start to feel the need to eat again. One of your body's triggers for hunger is your blood glucose level. A slow and sustained release of blood glucose that you get with a low-GI diet keeps blood glucose levels on an even keel, and levels tend not to drop to the hunger point for three to four hours, compared to only a couple of hours with a high-GI diet.

The insulin and blood sugar link

Insulin is a clever little hormone because it allows glucose to enter certain cells of the body, such as the muscles, which need ready fuel to produce energy. If the sugar is not required immediately, insulin helps sugar enter the liver, where it gets stored as glycogen, which acts as a reserve when you need energy quickly. Any excess glucose that is still lurking when immediate energy needs are satisfied and when glycogen stores are topped off, gets converted into fat, and again, insulin facilitates this process.

Of course, if the body is unable to produce enough insulin, such as in diabetes, your body has no way of stopping blood glucose levels from shooting very high and staying high for a long time. These high levels can lead to all kinds of damage to the body in the long term; in the short term, they can lead to coma and even death. For this reason, people with more severe type 2 diabetes or those with type 1 diabetes (where the body can't produce any insulin) have to have insulin shots or injections to deal with the rises in blood sugar that occur after meals.

The good news about a low-GI diet in this context is that if you're a diabetic requiring insulin shots, you probably don't need to take so much insulin if you follow a low-GI diet.

Achieving blood sugar control

The key to achieving blood sugar control is to eat foods that have a low GI rather than foods that have a high GI. The GI value of foods are classed as follows:

✔ **Low:** 55 or less

✔ **Medium:** 56 to 69

✔ **High:** 70 or more

Spaghetti and other low-GI foods don't cause a rapid rise and fall in blood glucose levels. Because your gut can't easily break down the sugar in low-GI food, it stays locked in for longer than the sugar in a high-GI food, such as a sugary drink. With low-GI foods, the sugar is slowly extracted from the food, so it only gets to trickle into the bloodstream as opposed to being dumped all at once. When you have PCOS, your body deals better with a steady trickle of sugar into the bloodstream rather than a rush so that you avoid high and low swings, which can wreak havoc in your body.

Testing food for its GI

Testing food for its GI value is an expensive and involved process and is only done in specialized research centers. So, not every single food with a GI value (which is any food that contains carbohydrate) has been tested, much to the frustration of avid low-GI followers! Here are the steps involved to determine the GI of a food:

1. **Ten or more healthy subjects consume a portion of the test food containing 50 grams of carbohydrate, and testers measure its effect on blood glucose levels over the next two-hour period.**

2. **On another occasion, the subjects consume a 50-gram portion of glucose (the reference food) and the testers measure its effect on blood glucose levels over the next two-hour period.**

3. **The GI is determined by dividing the area under the curve of the test food by the area under the curve of the reference food.**

   In the example shown in Figure 4-1, glucose is given a GI value of 100, whereas if the two-hour area under the blood sugar curve of the spaghetti were measured, it would be found to be 41 percent of that of the glucose. So, spaghetti is given a GI of 41.

   The final GI value is the average GI value of all ten subjects.

Low GI and PCOS

Because blood sugar levels don't shoot up but stay on an even keel on a low-GI diet, your body doesn't need to pump out lots of insulin to try to lower blood glucose levels. Therefore, levels of insulin in your blood stay low, providing that you generally continue to eat low GI. This habit can help you to lose weight more easily (after all, insulin promotes weight gain) and help to relieve many of your other symptoms of PCOS.

Low GI and diabetes

If you have PCOS and have developed diabetes that requires insulin shots, a low-GI diet can help you achieve the following:

- ✔ Better blood sugar control in the short and long term
- ✔ Less insulin required to control your blood sugar (and possibly eliminating the need for insulin altogether)
- ✔ Weight loss
- ✔ Lower risk of developing heart disease and other complications of diabetes

Low-fat vegan diets and glucose control

People who avoid meat appear to have better overall health, live longer, and suffer less heart disease and cancers than meat-eaters. A possible reason may be that non-meat-eaters are generally more aware of their diet and strive to eat a healthy diet and get more exercise. Another explanation may be that a meat-free diet tends to be high in fruit, vegetables, nuts, and seeds; higher in fiber; and lower in saturated fat. Avoiding meat also puts less of a strain on the kidneys and may help to offset kidney damage, which can occur if diabetes goes on for a long time without being adequately controlled.

A recent study of some 99 individuals, half of whom followed a vegan diet (free of *all* animal products — from meat and fish to dairy and eggs) and the rest of whom followed the type of diet advocated by the American Diabetes Association (ADA), produced some interesting results. After 22 weeks on these diets the researchers found that

- Forty-three percent of people following the vegan diet had been able to reduce their diabetic medication, compared to only 26 percent of those on the ADA diet.

- The overall diabetic control, measured by the amount of glucose circulating in the blood over a number of weeks, improved by twice as much in the vegan group as in the ADA group.

- Body weight decreased by 14 pounds in the vegan group compared to 7 pounds in the ADA group.

- Cholesterol levels decreased by 21.2 percent in the vegan group compared to 10.7 percent in the ADA group.

So, those following the vegan diet appeared to do twice as well as those following the ADA diet, but both groups achieved success. What this research shows is that, in addition to following a healthy, balanced diet, there also may be some merit in consuming more veggie meals or even meals that are just based on beans, legumes, grains, nuts, and seeds.

Remember: A vegan diet is tough for most people to follow, and if you do follow a vegan diet, you need to make sure that it contains sufficient nutrients, especially iron and calcium. But the good news is, you don't need to cut out animal products altogether. Have a few meat-free meals now and then, and use beans to provide your protein.

Spotting a low-GI carb

At first, distinguishing a low-GI carb from a high one may not seem that obvious. You also may be unsure at first about whether a food has a GI or not. Well, read on to find out.

Not all food has a GI value, because not all fo
carbohydrate content that is likely to have ar
cose levels. Foods that are pure meat, fish, or
carbs to speak of, so they can't be given a GI
trates examples of foods that do and don't ha

Table 4-1	Sample GI Values
Food	**GI Value**
White baguette	95
Chocolate puffed wheat cereal	77
Croissant	67
Cola	58
Sweet corn	53
Carrots	47
Apple	38
Chickpeas, boiled	28
Peanuts	14
Cabbage	No GI value
French beans	No GI value
Zucchini	No GI value
Nuts	No GI value

In order for a food to have a GI value, enough of it must be eaten to provide 50 grams of carbohydrate. Some foods are so low in carbs that eating an amount that provides 50 grams of carbs is impossible. Therefore, some vegetables (especially green vegetables) and nuts may not be given a GI value.

You can quickly get to know which carbs are low GI or not, but they're hard to identify in the raw without understanding a few rules about what makes a food low GI. Bottom line to remember: Some foods take longer to break down and release their sugar content into the bloodstream than other foods do.

The type of starch in food

Starch is a storage form of glucose found in plant foods. Starch is composed of hundreds or thousands of glucose molecules that are strung together in chains.

Two main kinds of starch are present in plant foods: amylopectin and amylose. When these starches are digested, their glucose molecules are liberated and absorbed, causing a rise in blood sugar. However, because of the differences in their chemical structures, these two starches have very different effects on blood sugar.

- ✔ **Amylopectin** has a structure that resembles the branches of a tree, so it's easily attacked by digestive enzymes. Starchy foods that contain a high proportion of amylopectin — like baking potatoes and sticky, short-grain rice — are quickly digested and produce rapid rises in blood sugar levels.

- ✔ **Amylose,** on the other hand, consists of a long, straight chain of tightly packed glucose molecules that resists digestion. Foods high in amylose — such as new potatoes and basmati rice — are absorbed more slowly and have lower glycemic indexes.

Cooking method

Cooking can increase the GI of a food. During cooking and baking, the starches in foods like grains, pastas, breads, and muffins absorb water. This causes the starch granules to swell and rupture, a process known as *gelatinization*. Gelatinized starch is readily attacked by digestive enzymes and very quickly digested and absorbed. Bread has a high GI partly because the starch in the finely ground flour used to make bread is easily gelatinized. And soft, overcooked pasta has a higher GI than firm, al dente pasta because the overcooked pasta absorbs more water during cooking.

Degree of food processing

Highly processed foods are digested faster and usually have a higher GI value. New technologies for processing grains — such as explosion puffing, extruding, and flaking — have been developed, and these tend to start to break down the starch in that grain and raise its GI value. For example, instant oat cereal has a higher GI than oatmeal.

Fibrous coat

An intact fibrous coat, such as that on grains and legumes, acts as a physical barrier to digestive enzymes, so it slows down the digestive process, which lowers a food's GI.

A food's fat content

Foods with a higher fat content have a lower GI rating. A high fat content means that food has to stay in the stomach longer, so the whole digestive process is slowed down. However, you shouldn't use this as an excuse to eat fatty meals, or you're going to end up gaining more weight and increase your risk of developing heart disease and certain cancers.

The advantage gained by slightly lowering the GI of a food or a meal by upping fat intake definitely does not outweigh the health gains from keeping fat intake down!

A food's fiber content

High fiber content in a food tends to slow the rate at which the starch in the food can be broken down. The two types of fiber are *soluble* (found in oats, beans, fruits, and vegetables) and *insoluble* (found in cereal fibers such as bran). Soluble fiber lowers the GI best.

Beans and legumes have a low GI because their starch content is wrapped in a fibrous shell, which the digestive enzymes take a while to get through. Research has shown that in addition to its effect on GI, a high-fiber meal seems to have a benefit that continues through to the next meal, causing a more even blood sugar control compared to a meal that had the same GI but lower fiber content.

The acid content of a food

When acid is present in a food, it slows your digestion. The naturally occurring acids in fruits, as well as the acids in fermented foods such as yogurt, buttermilk, and sourdough bread, slow the rate of digestion and contribute to the low GI of these foods. Likewise, adding just 4 teaspoons of vinegar or lemon juice to a meal can lower the GI of the meal by about 30 percent. For this reason, using vinegar and lemon juice to flavor foods can be a way to lower the GI of your diet.

The type of sugar present

You may be surprised to discover that, with the exception of glucose (GI = 100), most sugars have low to moderate GI values. Fructose, the sugar that occurs naturally in fruits, is very slowly absorbed, giving it a GI of only 23. Lactose, the sugar naturally present in milk and dairy products, has a GI of 46. This is one reason why most fruits and dairy products have such low glycemic indexes. Sucrose, a combination of equal parts fructose and glucose, has a GI of 65. The fact that sucrose is part fructose is one reason why many sweets have a moderate GI.

Finding resources for GI values

Here are some websites that allow free access to GI values:

✔ www.glycemicindex.com: This site comes highly recommended for being clear, thorough, and reliable. The site calls itself "The Official Website of the Glycemic Index and GI Database" and is run by the University of Sydney. In addition to having an extensive database of GI values, it has other information about GI, the GI diet, and the most up-to-date research on GI.

✔ www.mendosa.com/gilists.htm: This site is a searchable table of over 2,400 foods. The entries represent a true international effort of testing around the world.

✔ www.gilisting.com: This site has an online glycemic index database and some diet tips.

✔ www.shaklee.com/pws/library/products/wm_gi_g1_ tables.pdf: This is a PDF file (which you can search) containing an exam- ple of a GI breakfast meal makeover.

If you're looking for a book you can carry with you, try *The Low GI Shopper's Guide to GI Values 2011: The Authoritative Source of Glycemic Index Values for Nearly 1,500 Foods,* by Dr. Jennie Brand-Miller and Kaye Foster-Powell (De Capo Lifelong Books).

If you were to make a banana cake without sugar, the ripe bananas and flour in the cake would give it an overall GI of 55. However, adding sugar to the cake in the form of sucrose brings down the average GI of the cake to 47!

However, just because sugar in the form of sucrose or fructose doesn't have a high GI doesn't mean that you can add it liberally to everything. Pure sugar provides calories and no other real nutri- ents. That's why sugar is said to provide empty calories — it helps pile on the pounds without providing any other nutritional value. Far better to save those calories for something nutritious!

Meal Planning the Low-GI Way

Armed with the basics, you need to get down to the nitty-gritty: How do you throw a low-GI meal together?

When you have a meal you need to remember two things in order to ensure that your meal is low GI:

✔ You need to base your meal on a carbohydrate food.

✔ You need to make sure that the carb you're basing it on is low GI.

To help you along the way, here's a list of some examples of low-GI starches you may want to base each meal on:

✔ **Breakfast:** Oat-based breakfast cereal; barley-based breakfast cereal; cereal high in bran; cereal with plenty of dried fruits, nuts, and seeds; multigrain toast

✔ **Midmorning snack:** A handful of nuts, berries, or another low-GI snack

✔ **Lunch:** Whole-grain tortillas, flatbread, whole-grain cracker with seeds, sweet potato, whole-grain bread, rye bread, sourdough bread, pasta, cooked cold potato (for example, as potato salad)

✔ **Midafternoon snack:** A piece of low-GI fruit, such as an apple or pear

✔ **Dinner:** Brown rice, legumes (peas, beans, or lentils), noodles, pasta, sweet potatoes, new potatoes (boiled), a side salad with a vinegar dressing or balsamic vinegar

Constructing a meal

Many of your meals are going to be based on one starchy component; for example, in a traditional meal of meat, two vegetables, and potato, the potato is the starchy component. So, for meals made of just one carb-containing food, if that food has a low GI, the overall meal is low GI. However, if the meal is made up of more than one starchy food, the GI of that meal is the weighted average contribution of each carb (*weighted* meaning that the carb that is providing the greatest quantity exerts its GI effect more).

This weighting means that you can balance out a high-GI carb in a meal with a lower one, ending up with a meal that has a medium GI. An example is a baked potato with baked beans. Baked potatoes have a high GI, whereas baked beans have a low GI. If you eat them together, you end up with a medium-GI meal (providing you're using more than just a small amount of beans!).

Adding plenty of vegetables or a salad also lowers the overall GI of a meal, because they're low-GI foods.

A note on limiting carb intake

Although not eating starch or carbs in general may help to keep blood sugar levels down, it isn't the answer.

A low-carb diet means that the majority of your calories come from fat and protein. This kind of diet brings a risk of heart disease, increasing your blood pressure and possibly leading to an impairment in kidney function. The latter is particularly the case if you have diabetes or insulin resistance and high blood pressure.

Such a diet also means that you produce a lot of *ketones,* which are substances produced in elevated amounts when you're trying to metabolize a lot of fat in your diet as opposed to carbohydrate. Ketones can make you feel slightly nauseous and also make your breath smell nasty! If you're trying to get pregnant on a ketone-producing diet, you should be aware that ketones in the mother's bloodstream have been found to be toxic to the unborn child.

Other Advice for Healthy Eating

No one likes rules and rigidity, especially to do with food. However, you do need to keep a few things in mind when following a low-GI diet:

- ✔ When you eat a carb, make sure that it's a low-GI one.

- ✔ If finding a low-GI food is difficult, or if you just want a change occasionally, go for a medium-GI food.

- ✔ For a special occasion (or if you've gone to a friend's house for a meal and you don't want to be rude), eating an occasional high-GI food isn't going to hurt too much.

To keep your diet healthy *and* low GI, follow these tips:

- ✔ **For drinks, have a diet soft drink, tea or coffee (in moderation), or a low-cal hot chocolate.** If you need to sweeten your hot drink, use artificial sweeteners — this saves on empty calories. Also, avoid drinking more than one or two alcoholic beverages a day, and mostly stick to dry wines or spirits with diet mixers.

✔ **Aim for a minimum of five portions of fr**
daily. Opt for fresh or frozen, not canned.

✔ **Avoid adding salt to foods and reduce the c**
high-salt foods.

✔ **Don't eat too much protein foods, such as meat,**
poultry, and cheese. Two servings of these a day is ...e. If you're
a vegetarian, use soy products or peas, beans, and lentils as protein alternatives. In fact, these foods are nutritious and low in fat,
so they're great to eat even if you aren't vegetarian.

✔ **Keep your fat intake down.** Avoid frying your food, and swap
saturated fats (such as butter, lard, cakes, biscuits, and pastries) with polyunsaturated or monounsaturated fats and oils.
Avoid trans fats; if you see *partially hydrogenated* on the label,
that's a food to avoid.

✔ **Try to have three servings of dairy foods a day to ensure**
that you get enough calcium. A serving is one small container
of yogurt, ⅔ cup of milk, or 1 ounce of cheese.

✔ **Get plenty of fiber in your diet.** Fiber may give an added
boost to blood sugar control over and above the effect of GI
alone. Try to get between 25 grams and 35 grams of fiber per
day; most Americans consume only around 11 grams of fiber
per day!

✔ **If you need to lose weight, watch your portion sizes and**
how often you eat, even if you're eating low-GI foods.

✔ **Allow yourself one treat a day, such as a small scoop of**
ice cream or a low-GI bakery item, like a muffin or a small
piece of pound cake.

✔ **Don't take nutritional supplements or follow alternative**
therapies without guidance from a health worker who is
professionally qualified, such as a doctor or dietitian. For
more on alternative therapies, turn to Chapter 8.

British nutritionists have devised a pictorial representation of the
components of a healthy diet, called the Balance of Good Health,
shown in Figure 4-2.

The following sections give you some other guidance in order to
make sure that your diet is both balanced and low GI.

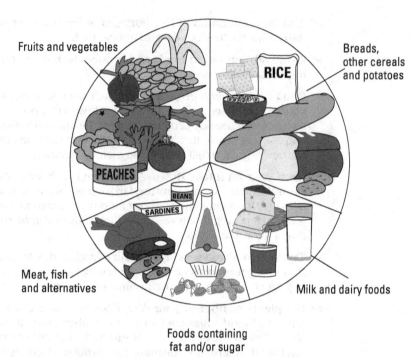

Figure 4-2: Balancing food types and portion sizes keeps your diet on track.

Do you ever need high-GI foods?

If you're a fairly serious athlete, during the course of whatever activity you're doing, your body uses up all its reserves of energy. This reserve is stored as glycogen, which is basically just a nice, compact form of glucose that's fairly easy for your body to access when needed. The majority of glycogen is stored in the liver; some is stored in muscle tissue.

However, a big match, a long run, or any energetic activity conducted for an hour or so is going to use up this glycogen store. For an athlete, restoring this store as soon as possible is essential, because you never know when you may need it again, and you can be prone to bouts of exhaustion without it.

The quickest way to restore this glycogen store is to get some glucose delivered into the bloodstream pronto. And what's the best way of doing that? Well, eating some high-GI food as quickly after the match as you can. But you don't want something fatty because that slows down the digestion and adds a lot of calories.

Energy drinks such as Gatorade, Powerade, Endurox, or Cytomax do the job. Look for drinks that contain sodium (because they're absorbed faster) and a small amount of protein (which may improve hydration after a workout).

Pay attention to portion size

Just because you're eating mostly low-GI foods and following the basic principles outlined in this chapter, doesn't guarantee weight loss. You may still be eating a lot of food or eating food too often. No amount of low-GI eating is going to help you keep your energy intake down if you end up eating large portions and eating too frequently. If the total number of calories you consume exceeds what your body needs, the excess calories just get stored as fat.

It may be helpful to keep an eye on how much food you serve up for yourself. If you like to fill your plate with food, just use a smaller plate.

Weigh out how much of these carb foods you normally serve yourself and then compare it to the normal portion sizes in Table 4-2. For a week, try to weigh out your carbs so that you only serve yourself a normal portion size. You'll soon get used to seeing how much a portion size looks on your plate. If you feel yourself slipping into giving yourself larger portions again, go back to weighing your carbs for a few days.

Table 4-2	Normal Portion Sizes for Low- to Medium-GI Foods
Food	**Normal Portion (Serving Size)**
All Bran cereal	1 small bowl (1½ ounces)
Oatmeal, made with water	1 small bowl (6 ounces)
Muesli	1 small bowl (2 ounces)
Basmati rice, uncooked	4 tablespoons (2 ounces)
Noodles, cooked	4 tablespoons (9 ounces)
Macaroni, cooked	4 tablespoons (9 ounces)
Spaghetti	4 tablespoons (9 ounces)
Pita bread	1 large (3 ounces)
Rye bread	1 slice (1 ounce)
Boiled potato	2 medium (7 ounces)

(continued)

Table 4-2 *(continued)*

Food	Normal Portion (Serving Size)
Sweet potato	1 medium (5 ounces)
Baked beans	1 small can (8 ounces)
Butter beans	4 tablespoons (5 ounces)
Chickpeas	4 tablespoons (6 ounces)
Red lentils	4 tablespoons (6 ounces)
Peanuts	1 small handful (2 ounces)
Apple juice	1 small glass (6 fluid ounces)
Orange juice	1 small glass (6 fluid ounces)

The food industry and GI

The food industry has not been blind to all the interest in GI. In Australia, everyone knows about GI, and many manufacturers and retailers label their foods with the GI value. This has been happening to a lesser extent in the United States and United Kingdom, although the biggest retail chain in the UK has been putting the GI value on its foods for a while. To be fair, manufacturers in the United States recognize that the real proven advantage of a low-GI diet is for diabetics and those with metabolic syndrome, insulin resistance, and PCOS. However, with growing obesity, that's likely to be an increasing number of consumers. Signs indicate that the low-GI diet may be great for people without any disease, too, but this evidence has dragged behind the evidence for its benefits in the aforementioned conditions.

Remember: If a food does carry a low-GI label, this doesn't guarantee it's healthy!

The other way that the food industry has been responding to the low-GI way of eating is through research and development: producing foods that are low GI. An example of this is in one of our biggest staples in the West — bread. Breads can now be manipulated to bring down the GI value by

✔ Adding different low-GI grains and/or seeds

✔ Enclosing the grain kernels so they break down slower

✔ Using sourdough fermentation

✔ Adding acid

✔ Using cereals specially bred to have higher levels of the starch that breaks down slowly

✔ Upping the fiber level

You can now find plenty of low-GI breads on the market.

Don't give up if you go off the rails

Sticking to a low-GI regime is going to help you feel better in the long run because it helps control your PCOS symptoms. However, you can eat some high-GI foods once in a while without causing irreversible damage! If you get the chance, you can limit the effect of eating a high-GI food in the following ways:

- ✔ In the same meal, try to have a low-GI food such as yogurt, milk, or low-GI beans as an accompaniment.

- ✔ Have plenty of veggies or salad with your meal.

- ✔ If you have an afternoon snack, make it a low-GI food, such as a piece of fruit.

- ✔ Have something acidic with your food, such as vinegar or lemon juice.

- ✔ Make sure that your next meal or snack is a low-GI one.

The GI effect of low-GI meals tends to build up. In other words, if you have a low-GI breakfast, it tends to have a lasting effect through to lunch and even dinner. Even if you have a high-GI lunch, the effect on your blood glucose level isn't going to be as bad as if you had no breakfast or a high-GI breakfast. Although not as pronounced as a low-GI breakfast, other meals may be able to have a continuous effect to the next meal as well.

Like any diet, don't let one meal or one day's failure set you back. After any relapse, just start fresh again as if you had never failed!

Not all low-GI foods are created equal

Just because a food has a low GI doesn't necessarily make it the healthiest choice. Table 4-3 lists some low-GI foods that may not be the wisest choice due to the fact that they may be high in fat, salt, or both. The right-hand column offers some advice as to whether these foods should be limited to once a day, once a week, or once a month.

If the table says you can have a product once a day, week, or month, don't have this and all the other products listed once a day, week, or month. You can have one treat *or* another!

Table 4-3		Low-GI Foods to Limit
Food	*GI*	*Recommended Frequency of Consumption*
Banana cake	47	Once a week
Chocolate cake with chocolate frosting	38	Once a month
Sponge cake	46	Once a week
Apple muffins	44	Once a week (daily if you make your own low-fat version)
Chocolate brownie	23	Once a week
Cookie	55	Once a day
Ice cream, premium, vanilla	38	Once a week (daily if you make your own with low-fat milk and fruit)
Custard with sugar	43	Once a week (daily if you make your own with low-fat milk)
Frozen yogurt	33	Once a day as a dessert
Full-fat yogurt	36	Once a week (daily if you opt for low-fat yogurt that is sugar free)
Milk shake/flavored milk	35	Once a month (daily if made with reduced-fat milk and artificial sweeteners)
Corn chips	42	Once a week
Potato chips	54	Once a week
Salted peanuts	14	Once a week (a small handful daily if unsalted)
Peanut M&M's	33	Once a week
White chocolate	44	Once a week
Plain or milk chocolate	43	Once a week
Hazelnut chocolate spread	33	Once a month
Vegetable pizza, takeout	49	Once a month (daily if you make your own with a low-fat base and topping)

Sorting the GI from the GL

You may have heard of the low-GL diet and wondered what it's all about. This diet is basically another way of trying to ensure that what you eat doesn't send your blood sugars shooting up too quickly. It involves another layer of complication and explanation, which is unnecessary; just counting the GI is fine. However, because many people do talk about the glycemic load (GL) of a food, it's only fair to give you some sort of explanation.

As explained elsewhere in this chapter, the glycemic index (GI) is a numerical system of measuring how much of a rise in circulating blood sugar a carbohydrate triggers — the higher the GI, the greater the blood sugar response. So, a low-GI food causes a small rise, whereas a high-GI food triggers a dramatic spike. The GL is a relatively new way to assess the impact of carbohydrate consumption that takes the glycemic index into account, but also takes into account the amount of the food — the quality and quantity of carbohydrate — that you consume. To work out the GL, you have to know how much carbohydrate is in a serving of a particular food.

Glycemic load is calculated this way:

$$GL = GI \div 100 \times (\text{total carbs} - \text{dietary fiber})$$

A GL of 20 or more is high, a GL of 11 to 19 is medium, and a GL of 10 or less is low.

The drawback of the GL system is that low-GL foods are likely to be low GI simply because they're low carb. What this means is that if you were to try to follow a low-GL diet alone, it might not be the healthiest way to eat because it might be high in fat and protein and low in carbs.

The key to getting the best blood glucose response is to eat more low-GI carbohydrates, not to eat less carbohydrates. GL doesn't distinguish slow carb from low carb; you need the carbs, but the slow-release kind, not the ones that rush in!

Fortunately you don't need to go to the extent of working out the GL of your food, which just adds another layer of complexity you don't need. Take a look at *The GL Diet For Dummies,* by Nigel Denby and Sue Baic (Wiley), if you want to know more.

Chapter 5

Shedding the Extra Load

• •

In This Chapter

▶ Determining how much you need to lose

▶ Losing weight sensibly and effectively

▶ Combining the low-GI diet with a weight loss diet

▶ Controlling cravings

▶ Assembling a dieting tool box

▶ Bouncing back from setbacks

• •

*N*o doubt about it: PCOS is associated with being overweight. More than half of patients with PCOS are obese. Recent research has also shown that if you're overweight, your chances of having PCOS are around five times higher than if you are normal weight.

This chapter goes into detail on how to lose weight if you have PCOS and how to overcome certain obstacles that come your way. If you have PCOS, you're likely to need to watch your weight quite carefully, if not actually reduce it by a certain amount. You discover in this chapter how to maintain the low-GI diet (see Chapter 4), but tailor it to weight loss as well. This chapter also looks at coping with hunger and cravings, which are particularly common if you live with PCOS.

Deciding How Much to Lose

Your dietitian or doctor may have already given you a goal weight to reach, or you may want to set your own target. You can find the most scientific and sensible approaches for setting targets in this section.

If you have a lot of weight to lose, aim for a target of around 5 pounds at a time.

Body mass index

The healthy weight range is based on a measurement known as the body mass index (BMI), determined from your weight and height.

You can find your BMI by going to www.nhlbisupport.com/bmi and entering your height and weight into the BMI calculator.

If you'd rather do the math yourself (have a calculator ready!), follow these three simple steps:

1. **Measure your height in inches and multiply the figure by itself.**

   For example, if you're 5'6" tall, that's 66 inches. So, you multiply $66 \times 66 = 4{,}356$.

2. **Measure your weight in pounds and multiply by 703.**

   For example, if you're 160 pounds, you multiply $160 \times 703 = 112{,}480$.

3. **Divide the answer in Step 2 by the answer in Step 1.**

   Using our running example, $112{,}480 \div 4{,}356 = 25.8$. That's your BMI.

Now turn to Table 5-1 to determine what your BMI means.

Table 5-1	Recommended BMI Chart
BMI	*Classification*
18.4 or less	Underweight
18.5 to 24.9	Ideal
25 to 29.9	Overweight
30 to 39.9	Obese
40 or more	Very obese

The BMI measurement may be inaccurate if you're an athlete or very muscled (muscle weighs more than fat), because it can push you into a higher BMI category despite having a healthy level of body fat. The measurement is also not accurate for women who are pregnant or breast-feeding, or people who are frail.

Health professionals are now also realizing that some people can have an ideal BMI but still be at risk for developing obesity-type symptoms because they carry too much weight around the middle. Women with PCOS may fall into this category; your BMI may be in the ideal range, but you still may develop insulin resistance because of the excess weight you carry around your tummy. So, your BMI may not be the ideal measure for you to determine your ideal weight if you have PCOS. Still, if your BMI is 25 or above, and you aren't an elite athlete, pregnant, or breast-feeding, you should lose weight.

BMI is only one guide in determining your overall health. Waist measurement, body fat level, blood pressure, cholesterol, physical activity, not smoking, and the healthiness of your diet are also important. You need to get the whole picture.

Waist circumference

The measurement of waist circumference provides information about the distribution of body fat and is a measure of risk for conditions such as diabetes. Experts now know that people who carry their excess fat centrally (around the tummy area) are more likely to suffer the consequences of being overweight.

The correct position for measuring waist circumference is midway between the upper hipbone and the lower rib. Place the tape measure around the abdomen at the level of this midway point, breathe out, and take a reading when the tape is snug but doesn't push down the skin.

In practice if you're very overweight, it may be difficult for you to accurately find those bony landmarks, in which case placing the tape at the level of the belly button is recommended.

For women, a waist circumference measure of over 31½ inches indicates an increased risk of developing heart disease, diabetes, blood pressure, and other related diseases.

Waist circumference can be used as an additional measure of progress with weight loss, especially because physical activity can help you lose inches off your waist, even before you lose much weight.

Apples and pears

If you have too much weight around your middle, you may be described by some health professionals as having an "apple" shape and told that you have an increased risk of developing heart disease and diabetes. When men gain weight, they often gain it round the middle, which is often referred to as a "beer belly." When women gain weight, they don't tend to put it on around the middle as much as men do — unless, that is, they have PCOS. Normally, women are offered some protection against heart disease by not developing an apple shape like men. Unfortunately this protection can be lost if you have PCOS. Post-menopause, women also tend to put on weight in this area, which increases their risk of developing diabetes and heart disease.

If you tend to gain weight around your hips, you have a "pear" shape. This tends to be a less risky place to gain weight as far as heart disease and related health risks are concerned. Someone who has an apple shape faces greater health risks than someone who has a pear shape, even if they're both overweight to the same degree.

To determine whether you're an apple or a pear, measure your waist circumference, about an inch above your belly button. Then measure your hip circumference, around the widest area of your lower body. Divide your waist measurement by your hip measurement. If the result is 0.8 or lower, you're a pear. If it's larger than 0.8, you're an apple.

Before You Begin to Trim

You're probably already aware that it tends to be harder to lose weight if you have PCOS. No one is exactly sure why, but it may be a combination of:

- ✔ Generally having a lowered metabolic rate so that you just burn your fat that much slower.

- ✔ Always feeling hungry and more prone to food cravings so that cutting down on your food intake is harder for you.

- ✔ The higher circulating insulin levels may mean that you have a greater tendency to store excess fuel as fat, rather than burning it up.

Although losing weight is never easy, following the guidelines outlined in the next sections can make the process easier — or at least a little less painful.

Rule #1: Lose weight slowly

Slow weight loss is better than rapid weight loss if you have PCOS, unless of course your doctor has told you that losing weight is an urgent need for you. Losing 1 to 2 pounds per week is ideal. This weight loss is achievable, even if you struggle to diet. Weight lost slowly is also less likely to be regained and you're less likely to go into that yo-yo situation where you lose weight, regain it, lose it again, and so on.

Yo-yo dieting is thought to be harmful, and the regained weight is more likely to be fat, so after a few repeating cycles, you have a lower muscle mass and a higher fat mass than someone of the same weight as you who never dieted.

Rule #2: Pick the best of the diet bunch

Instead of working out your own diet and checking that all the sums add up for the calorie values (and that your fat and sugar levels aren't out of balance), you may want to pick a weight-loss diet "off the shelf" or see a dietitian and get some guidance. With any diet plan you choose, check that it's balanced and states how many calories it provides.

Commercial weight-loss programs such as Weight Watchers can be very helpful, but tell them you have PCOS and want to follow a low-GI approach. Most programs are familiar with this concept and should be able to offer some positive advice.

Web-based diet organizations and forums can be very helpful — some even offer low-GI diets specifically. You may have to pay to join, but they're often cheaper than going to in-person meetings. Most sites have a members' chat room. Again, before joining check out that the diet advice is sound and follows the guidance given in this book.

Here are some basic guidelines to follow to make sure that you don't pick a dud diet:

- ✔ Avoid diets that claim huge weight losses in a short space of time.

- ✔ If you plan to follow a diet for longer than a month, around 1,500 calories per day is a good level of intake. For shorter time periods, when you have less than 15 pounds to lose, you can drop to 1,300 calories. Never go below 1,200 calories.

- ✔ Avoid diets that tell you to avoid certain foods or groups of foods.

- ✔ Avoid diets that advocate only a narrow range of foods.

- ✔ Make sure that the diet isn't a low-carbohydrate diet.

- ✔ Check whether the diet plan is also adaptable to a low-GI way of eating.

Although some procedures and drugs make you appear to have lost weight, these are only temporary solutions due to water loss. After a day or so, providing you're drinking normally, the weight goes back on because you haven't lost fat. The following techniques make you lose water but don't provide a real loss in fat mass:

- ✔ Body wraps

- ✔ Saunas or steam rooms

- ✔ Diuretic pills, including "natural" herbal diuretics

You also may see claims that certain natural chemicals can make you lose weight, including:

- ✔ Caffeine and other stimulants

- ✔ Green tea extract

- ✔ Conjugated linoleic acid, a type of fat naturally present in small amounts in dairy foods and that you can buy as a supplement

Some evidence suggests that these substances can speed up metabolism, but the evidence is not yet conclusive, and the extra calories you burn off by consuming these substances is minimal.

Stimulants such as caffeine are not well tolerated by everyone and can lead to high blood pressure and other health problems.

Following a Low-GI and Weight-Loss Diet

The theory behind weight loss is very simple:

- ✔ If energy in equals energy out, weight remains stable.

- ✔ If energy in is greater than energy out, weight gain occurs.

- ✔ If energy in is less than energy out, weight loss occurs.

That's the theory, but in practice reducing your intake and increasing your output is painful, psychologically if not physically! The task becomes even trickier if you have PCOS. Ideally, you need to think about low-GI requirements as well as calorie requirements.

You don't have to lose a lot of weight to start to see the benefits in terms of your PCOS symptoms. If you're overweight, even losing 5 percent of your body weight leads to the following beneficial changes:

- ✔ A decrease in insulin resistance leading to a beneficial lowering of circulating insulin levels.

- ✔ An improvement in the regularity of your periods; missing periods may well return with even this small weight loss.

- ✔ A lowering of testosterone level leading to the reduction of unwanted facial hair and acne.

- ✔ More general health benefits, such as lowering your cholesterol levels and reducing your risk of developing diabetes and heart disease.

Combining low GI and low calories

For maximum health benefit, and particularly if you have weight to lose, a low-GI diet alone just doesn't cut it. You also need to reduce calories. (Check out Chapter 4 for more information on the low-GI diet.)

Starchy foods in your diet should be low-GI starches. You also may need to avoid certain foods that, although low in calories, aren't low GI, as well as low-GI foods that aren't low in calories. Table 5-2 lists foods to avoid.

Table 5-2   Low- and High-GI Foods to Avoid

Low/Moderate-Calorie but High-GI Foods	Low-GI but High-Calorie Foods
Cornflakes	Full-fat milk
Puffed wheat	Chocolate
Puffed rice	Fruit cake
White rice	Sponge cake
Rice cakes	Ice cream

(continued)

Table 5-2 *(continued)*

Low/Moderate-Calorie but High-GI Foods	Low-GI but High-Calorie Foods
White flour crackers	Creamy sauces
Bagels	Whole milk yogurt
French bread	Tortilla or corn chips
Baked potatoes	
Meringue	
Sorbet	

When you have PCOS, you have a tendency to feel very hungry, quite often. Some of this hunger may be due to fluctuating glucose levels. A low-GI diet can help to stabilize hunger by reducing blood sugar fluctuations. Having a regular meal pattern also helps to prevent extreme hunger, and this pattern may involve having some small low-GI snacks between meals, too.

Several research studies show that a low-GI diet can lead to weight loss and increased feelings of satiety. However, other studies have failed to prove this, so to a certain extent, the jury is still out. The reason for following a low-GI diet when you have PCOS is to bring circulating insulin levels down and alleviate some of the symptoms. The fact that a low-GI diet may help with weight loss is an added bonus!

Knowing what you need: Daily recommended amounts

You need a certain amounts of nutrients every day for a balanced and healthy diet. In general, by eating 2,000 calories a day, you would probably not lose or gain weight, unless you're exceptionally active or exceptionally sedentary. If you have a lot of weight to lose, you may be able to lose it by cutting a couple hundred calories a day. However, a good general rule is to cut your calorie intake by about 500 calories per day to lose weight.

Table 5-3 shows the recommended daily amounts for weight maintenance and for weight loss.

Table 5-3   Weight Maintenance and Weight Loss

Nutrient	Weight Maintenance	Weight Loss
Calories	2,000	1,500
Total fat	70 grams	50 grams
Saturated fat	20 grams	15 grams
Total sugars	90 grams	70 grams

Armed with a calorie counter guide and by looking at the nutritional label, you can see whether a food is likely to fit into your overall calorie-controlled diet. For example, consider a hamburger that contains 600 calories, 40 grams of fat, and 15 grams of saturated fat. Is it so desirable that you want to blow nearly half your calorie allowance for the day on it, plus over half your total fat and all your saturated fat limit?

Getting the right portion sizes

When following a 1,500-calorie plan, in order for it to be balanced and stay within your calorie limit, use the recommended number of portions outlined in Table 5-4.

Table 5-4   Recommended Portions of Food on a 1,500-Calorie Diet

Food	Daily Portions
Breads, cereals, potatoes, rice, pasta	6
Meat, fish, eggs, legumes, and nuts	2
Milk and dairy foods	3
Vegetables	At least 3
Fruit	3
Oils, dressings, and spreads	3
Extras, such as snacks and alcohol	1

So that you know roughly what one portion equates to, use the following guidelines:

✓ **Breads, potatoes, cereals, rice, pasta:**

- Small bowl (about 3 heaped tablespoons) breakfast cereal or oatmeal

- One medium slice of bread, mini pita, or small tortilla

- Half a medium pita, tortilla, wrap, or roll

- Two new potatoes or one medium potato (including sweet potatoes)

- ½ cup cooked pasta or 1 ounce uncooked pasta

- ⅓ cup cooked rice or barley or 1 ounce uncooked rice or barley

✓ **Meat, chicken, fish, eggs, seeds, and nuts:**

- 3 to 4 ounces cooked lean meat or oily fish (uncooked weights are about a quarter heavier)

- 6 ounces white fish or seafood

- 6 ounces meat-based tomato-type sauce such as Bolognese or chili

- Two eggs (but avoid more than six eggs per week if your cholesterol is high)

- 5 tablespoons cooked beans, lentils, baked beans, or tofu

- Just under 1½ ounces nuts, seeds, or nut butter

- 3 ounces reduced-fat hummus

✓ **Milk and dairy foods:**

- 1 cup skim milk or ⅔ cup 2 percent milk or fortified soymilk

- A small container of low-fat yogurt

- 1 ounce cheese

- 2 ounces low-fat cream cheese

- 2 heaped tablespoons cottage cheese

✓ **Vegetables:**

- 3 heaping tablespoons any type of vegetable (fresh, frozen, or canned)

- Bowl of salad

✔ **Fruits:**

- 1 medium piece of fruit, such as apple, orange, or pear
- 1 cup berries or grapes
- 2 small pieces of fruit, such as Mandarin oranges or plums
- 1 large slice of fruit such as melon or pineapple
- 3 tablespoons canned or stewed fruit in juice
- 6 fluid ounces of unsweetened fruit juice
- 1 tablespoon dried fruit

✔ **Oils, dressings, and spreads:**

- 1 teaspoon oil, spread, margarine, or mayonnaise
- 2 teaspoons low-fat spread or salad dressing
- 1 tablespoon sour cream
- 2 tablespoons fat-free dressing

✔ **Extras (around 100 calories each):**

- Two fruit servings
- One dairy serving, such as low-fat yogurt
- 1 slice of low-GI bread with low-fat spread
- 2 low-GI crackers with 2 ounces tuna or thinly spread peanut butter or low-fat cream cheese
- 1 ounce nuts and raisins
- 1 small cereal bar or mini chocolate bar
- A small bag of snacks such as reduced chips that don't exceed 100 calories
- A small glass of wine, half a pint of beer, or an ounce of hard alcohol with a low-cal mixer

Don't forget to have at least six to eight glasses of water or other low-cal liquids throughout the day.

You can have the following drinks and not need to count them as part of your diet:

✔ Water, including still or sparkling mineral water and flavored low-calorie still or sparkling waters

✔ Diet soft drinks and carbonated drinks

✔ Herbal teas

✔ Tea and coffee

Here's some stuff that you don't have to count — you can use these to spice up your food:

✔ Lemon or lime juice

✔ Vinegar

✔ Herbs and spice

✔ A few capers or olives

✔ Boullion cube (but watch the sodium intake — they're quite salty)

✔ Soy or teriyaki sauce (but not too much because these are salty, too)

✔ Hot pepper sauce, such as Tabasco or Worcestershire sauce

✔ Mustard

✔ Tomato purée

✔ A splash of wine (If used in cooking, the alcohol — and most carbs — evaporate.)

Although you need to decide how you spread these portions around in a day, Table 5-5 offers a suggested approach.

Table 5-5   Spread of Portions for Each Meal

Food	Breakfast	Lunch	Main Meal	Snacks
Breads, cereals, potatoes, rice, pasta	1	2	2	1
Meat, fish, eggs, legumes, and nuts		1	1	
Milk and dairy foods	1	1		1
Vegetables		1	3	
Fruit	1		1	1
Oils, dress-ings, and spreads	1	1	1	
Extras				1

Ready-to-eat meals

If you're out and about and you want to grab a quick sandwich for lunch, or a ready-made salad, go for one that's around 300 calories. If you don't have time to cook in the evening and you want to just heat up a microwaveable meal, choose one that's around 400 calories, but don't forget to serve it with plenty of extra veggies or a bowl of salad.

Food Addiction and Cravings

Cravings for starchy foods, such as bread, and sweet foods is common if you have PCOS, but nobody really knows why. One theory is that it's a similar craving that women with PMS get and is linked to changes in mood.

Overcoming cravings

Try the following to stop yourself from craving certain foods:

- ✔ Don't let yourself get extremely hungry because this often triggers a craving.

- ✔ Keep your blood sugar level on an even keel by following a low-GI diet.

- ✔ Don't skip meals. Incorporate snacks into your daily eating plan. Eating every few hours prevents you from getting too hungry before your next meal by preventing downward swings in blood sugar levels that can trigger a craving.

- ✔ Don't totally deny yourself foods that you really crave and love. If it's chocolate, have it after you've had a proper meal — and just have a little bit of some really good quality stuff.

- ✔ Get moving! Doing some exercise every day can help to normalize hunger and eating patterns.

- ✔ Don't diet or restrict your eating too strictly. Doing so is a common trigger for cravings. (The body can't stay in a state of denial for too long.)

Recognizing the dangers of bingeing

Bingeing is a form of *eating disorder*, a distorted pattern of thinking about food and behavior toward food. If you tend to binge on a regular basis, you may well have a preoccupation or obsession with food. You probably feel out of control as far as food is concerned. Women with PCOS are prone to binge and to have *bulimia* (which is where you binge, feel guilty, and try to purge yourself of what you've eaten — and then repeat the cycle again).

The binge cycle typically takes the following steps in PCOS: You start by feeling low in energy, mood, or self-esteem. To combat this feeling, you want to eat "comfort foods," such as bread or chocolate. You gain a short-term feeling of comfort (hence, the name "comfort foods"), but you also experience an increase in blood sugar levels and insulin levels, as well as hormone imbalance. And that leads back to feeling low in energy, mood, or self-esteem. And the cycle repeats itself.

The binge cycle must be broken, because the outcome of this repeated cycle is the following:

- ✔ Weight gain

- ✔ Bloating

- ✔ Further hormonal imbalances

- ✔ Increasingly low self-esteem

- ✔ Inappropriate compensatory practices such as missing meals

Six percent of women with PCOS have bulimia compared to 1 percent without PCOS. So, why are you more likely to have a binge eating disorder than someone without PCOS?

- ✔ **PCOS is a collection of disorders, including menstrual problems, an above-average weight, anxieties about fertility, and increased facial and body hair.** These symptoms are not something that make you feel particularly good about yourself. They can set up a situation where a normal relationship with food is not possible and bingeing becomes the way in which you deal with the emotional stress.

- ✔ **The fluctuating insulin levels that occur in PCOS and their subsequent effect on blood sugar levels can result in a feeling that you need to binge.** After bingeing, you may feel that you have to compensate somehow, so you attempt to starve yourself. The problem is that this sort of behavior, where bingeing is followed by starvation, can actually make insulin resistance worse.

Evidence is emerging that the desire to binge and the lack of a subsequent feeling of being satiated, which is commonly seen in PCOS, is due to hormone levels that are off-kilter. The body depends on these hormones to be at normal levels so that food intake can be kept on an even keel.

Some evidence suggests that cravings for sweet foods and a desire to binge on them is related to testosterone levels (which tend to be higher in women with PCOS). Testosterone may drive down the level of a hormone called *cholecystokinin,* which controls appetite. A lowered level of this hormone may predispose you to having an increased tendency to binge and gain weight, compared to women with a higher level. Further evidence exists that appetite regulation is impaired in women with PCOS due to the disruption of another appetite hormone, called *ghrelin.* Normally, ghrelin levels increase sharply before a meal, which stimulates hunger and drives food intake. As consumption of a meal progresses, the level of ghrelin falls and this helps the feeling of becoming satiated. However, in PCOS, this decline in ghrelin levels doesn't happen, or happens to a lesser extent, so the trigger to stop eating is reduced.

If you suspect that you truly have an eating disorder and/or that your bingeing behavior is out of control, you need some professional help from your primary-care doctor, who can refer you to a specialist and dietitian if necessary, as well as to a therapist.

Dieting Do's and Don'ts

No one has a surefire successful formula for dieting because the reasons people become overweight may be very different and the way that they respond to weight loss may be very different, too. However, this section offers a few tricks of the trade to help you reach your goal weight.

Keeping a diary

The diet diary is an essential tool for weight loss. It puts you in control, shows where things may be going wrong, and enables you to do some detective work on where and why you may be failing. The diary should include the following:

- The time you ate the food
- Where you ate it (for example, "Walking around the kitchen," "In front of the TV," or "At the dinner table with family")
- The food you ate
- How much you ate
- Your mood when you ate
- Whether you were hungry before you ate

To get the most benefit from a diet diary, heed these bits of advice:

✔ **Keep your diary with you at all times, and religiously write down what you eat as soon as you eat it.** Even the simple act of knowing that you have to write it all down can be enough to make you think twice about eating something you know you shouldn't. Plus, even with the best of intentions, you probably won't remember everything you've had throughout the day if you wait to jot it down in the evening, and that negates the usefulness of keeping the diary in the first place.

✔ **Try to spend some time analyzing your diary at the end of every week to see whether any patterns emerge.** If you've had a good week and lost weight, look back to see what you did to cause that weight loss. If you don't lose weight one week, go back through the diary to see whether you can spot where you went awry.

✔ **Keep the diary for at least a week or two.** If you worry that you're slipping back into old habits, you can look back on the good weeks to remind yourself that you *can* do it.

Recording your weight and body fat

Weight recording can be done in conjunction with your food diary. You can then match up your intake with what's happening to your weight and get a real feeling of cause and effect.

Weigh yourself only once a week because weight can fluctuate quite a lot on a daily basis. Try to do it at the same time of day and with the same type of clothes — or no clothes at all.

Consider investing in a scale that measures your body fat percentage. These scales are more expensive than ordinary scales, but they give you a better picture of what's going on in your body while you lose weight. If you're also embarking on an exercise program, you may find that you lose proportionally more body fat than you do weight. This is because some of your body fat is not simply being burned up, but is being used to make more muscle, and muscle weighs more than fat. Plus, if you work out, you may look more toned and slimmer than a woman of the same weight as you who doesn't work out.

Table 5-6 can help you to identify where you are healthwise with regard to your body fat percentage. You can see that as you get older, you're allowed a little more leeway with regards to how much body fat you can carry and still be in the healthy range.

Table 5-6 Recommended Body Fat Percentages for Women

Age	Underfat	Healthy	Overfat	Obese
16–17	Less than 16%	16%–30%	30%–35%	More than 35%
18	Less than 17%	17%–31%	31%–36%	More than 36%
19	Less than 19%	19%–32%	33%–37%	More than 37%
20–39	Less than 21%	21%–33%	34%–38%	More than 38%
40–59	Less than 23%	23%–34%	35%–40%	More than 40%

Arranging (rather than filling) your plate

When following a diet, you need to eat less energy-dense food (foods that provide a lot of calories in a small amount of the food) and try to fill up on foods that you can eat a lot of but that don't supply so many calories. Table 5-7 lists examples of foods with high, medium, and low energy densities.

Table 5-7	Energy Density of Foods
Energy Density	**Food**
High	Butter, oil, cheese, fatty meat, nuts, pastries, batter, full-fat dumplings, cake, biscuits, alcohol
Medium	Lean meat, poached or grilled fish, pasta, fruit juice, breakfast cereals, bread, rice
Low	Vegetables, fruit, beans, lentils

The foods with a high energy density provide lots of calories, so only eat a little of these in a day. Foods with a high energy density are usually high in fat; fatty foods are energy dense because fat has twice as many calories weight for weight as protein and carbs do. Foods with a low energy density, such as vegetables and legumes, should make up the largest part of your diet because they provide lots of vitamins and minerals but not many calories. These foods have a low energy density because they contain very little fat but usually contain quite a lot of water, which is, of course, calorie free.

When considering your dinner plate, plan to cover it with your dinner in the following healthy proportions (see Figure 5-1):

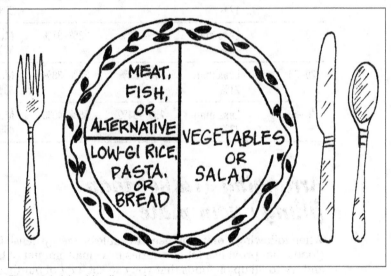

Figure 5-1: A healthy dinner plate.

- ✔ About half of your plate can be made up of vegetables or beans and lentils, which have a low energy density and fill you up without many calories.

- ✔ About a quarter of your plate can come from starchy foods such as pasta or rice, which have a medium energy density and provide low-GI carbs, help you feel full, and provide fiber and other nutrients.

- ✔ The last quarter of your plate can be the protein part of the meal, which has a medium energy density.

You can add to your plate a very small amount of foods with a high energy density, such as cheese, but do so with caution because they bump up your calories without your even noticing it.

If you like to fill your plate, or pile it high, and you have largish dinner plates, simply use a smaller plate so that even by filling your plate with food, you automatically get less!

Savoring every bite

In order for your body to register that it has had a meal and to feel satisfied with that, take time to fully appreciate what you put into your mouth. Try to be aware of every morsel you eat — you may begin to realize that you don't really want to be eating that particular food or at that particular time. You also may be more aware of when you're feeling full and be able to put your knife and fork down without having to finish everything on your plate.

Appreciating your food may help you eat less of it. Here are some tips on how to appreciate your food more:

- ✔ **Make an occasion of every mealtime.** Light the candles, add a vase of flowers, and use the good china.

- ✔ **Make sure you're eating food that's really tasty and nutritious.** Don't passively put any old junk food in your mouth.

- ✔ **Never eat standing up or walking around.** Ideally sit at a table when you're eating.

- ✔ **Use a plate (even if just having a snack) and utensils.**

- ✔ **Don't do anything else while you're eating, such as reading or watching television.** Exception: Engaging in conversation with your family and friends is encouraged. (After all, you can't talk with your mouth full!)

- ✔ **Eat slowly, savoring every mouthful and chewing it thoroughly.**

Planning your meals ahead of time

Never let yourself stumble up to a mealtime without knowing what you're going to have and without the ingredients or food at hand.

Plan out your week's menu and shop for that. You can do this on a daily basis if you have the opportunity to shop daily. Then you know exactly what ingredients you need and you don't end up buying extras (which you may be tempted to eat). Each morning, check what you're going to have for each meal. Then if a meal needs some pre-preparation, such as soaking beans or defrosting something, make sure you do that beforehand instead of leaving it until the actual mealtime.

If you don't plan ahead and you're ravenously hungry, you're going to be tempted to go for the first thing you can find (a bag of chips or a hunk of cheese) or send out for pizza.

Using healthy cooking methods

How healthy and how low-calorie your meal ends up being depends as much on the method you use to cook something as it does on the ingredients you use.

Healthy cooking methods don't need to be involved and drawn out; in fact, they can be hassle free. Here are some tips on how to prepare food the healthy way if you want to lose weight:

- ✔ Steam or microwave your vegetables so that they retain more nutrients and you don't add extra fat to them.

- ✔ Poach, boil, or scramble your eggs; don't fry them. Scrambled eggs can be made in the microwave using a little milk and black pepper whisked up with them. Only cook until just before they're set because they continue cooking after you remove them from the microwave.

- ✔ Grill or bake meat and pour away the fat.

- ✔ When cooking fairly fatty meat such as bacon or sausages, grill them and then place them on paper towels to blot away the remaining melted fat.

- ✔ When making a casserole or stew using meat with some fat on it, let it go cold, take off the solidified fat that appears on top, and then reheat.

- ✔ Don't use meat juices, which contain a lot of fat, when making gravy.

- ✔ Make your own salad dressing with just a little oil, herbs, lemon juice, and balsamic vinegar. This way, you can be sure that it's much lower in calories than store-bought dressing.

- ✔ Parboil Mediterranean vegetables and potatoes and roast in a little olive oil in the oven. You also can add minced garlic, pepper, and herbs.

Getting insight from people who have kept their weight off

The following tips have come from researching successful dieters who managed to keep their weight off. If it worked for them, it can work for you!

- ✔ **Getting an hour of physical activity a day helps to maintain weight loss.** If you can't manage this much, try to do at least half an hour a day.

- ✔ **Weigh yourself weekly.** If the weight seems to be creeping up again, take charge immediately before things get worse.

- ✔ **Continue to plan your meals.** This way, you know what you're going to eat at the next meal and you have the ingredients on hand.

- ✔ **Continue to follow your low-fat diet with your carbs coming from low-GI sources where possible.**

- ✔ **Have regular meals and snacks, and don't skip meals.**

- ✔ **Always eat breakfast.** It helps normalize your eating patterns for the rest of the day. (See the nearby sidebar, "The benefits of eating breakfast," for more.)

The National Weight Control Registry studies people who have managed to successfully maintain weight loss; they found that of those who were successful in maintaining their weight loss, only 9 percent managed to do so without doing some regular exercise.

The benefits of eating breakfast

If you think skipping breakfast is going to help you lose weight, think again! Studies show that breakfast, especially a cereal-based breakfast, is associated with better weight control.

An ongoing study by the National Weight Control Registry of people who have maintained weight loss of at least 30 pounds for more than a year shows that eating breakfast keeps people slimmer. Breakfast eaters tend to eat fewer calories, eat less saturated fat and cholesterol, and have better overall nutritional status than breakfast skippers. A Nielsen's National Eating Trends Survey showed that women who ate cereal on a regular basis weighed about 9 pounds less than those who ate cereal rarely or not at all.

When you skip breakfast, your metabolic rate tends to slow down and your blood sugar drops. As a result, you become hungry and have less energy. Without breakfast, you tend to want to snack in the morning, often on high-fat sweets, or to eat extra servings or bigger portions at lunch or dinner. However, when you eat breakfast, your body feels nourished and satisfied, making you less likely to overeat the rest of the day.

Eating a low-GI breakfast every day may reduce the risk for obesity and insulin resistance by as much as 35 percent to 50 percent.

Cereal bars have exploded in popularity. Although they're convenient and may satisfy your hunger, read the label. Even though they contain a variety of vitamins and other added nutrients, they often contain very little fiber and are loaded with as many calories as a chocolate bar!

When the Going Gets Tough

A couple of factors may tend to throw you off your diet: not losing any weight and giving in to temptation and falling off the wagon. But help is available for both these diet failure factors, as the following sections explain.

Figuring out why you're not losing weight

The scales at the end of the week may not always register a weight loss. Always keep a food diary when you've gone two weeks without losing weight because this record may help pinpoint what's happening.

In the following sections, we cover some common reasons you may not be losing weight.

You're kidding yourself

At the start of a diet, you're typically fired up and watching your food intake carefully. But after a while, you may start to get complacent and let some old habits creep back in, even though you may have convinced yourself that you're still on the diet. If your weight loss has slowed down or stopped, you need to check with your food diary whether you're really still eating as healthfully as you tell yourself you are.

You're already there

The reason that you're no longer losing weight or that the losses have slowed right down may be that you've lost enough. Use the following three checks to see where you are, and if you come out normal for two out of three, you've lost enough.

- ✔ Your body mass index (BMI) is 25 or less.

- ✔ Your waist circumference is 31½ inches or less.

- ✔ Your body-fat percentage is 21 percent to 33 percent if you're aged 20 to 39 or 23 percent to 34 percent if you're aged 40 to 59. (Refer to Table 5-6.)

You've gone too far

If you cut back too drastically on your calorie intake, or you exercise too intensively, you can actually hamper your weight loss. This reaction is because the body thinks it's in a state of emergency — either in a state of starvation or in a state when extreme endurance is required. Both of these factors tend to make the body store as many of the calories it's given as possible and stubbornly cling to its fat reserves.

Watch out for these key signs, which indicate that you're not giving your body nearly enough fuel:

- ✔ Frequent, sharp hunger pangs
- ✔ Mood swings
- ✔ Strongly fluctuating energy levels
- ✔ Dizziness
- ✔ Constant thoughts about food

Check your food diary — you need to take in around 1,500 calories a day and not skip meals. Also, check that you're having sufficient servings of each of the food groups listed in Table 5-5.

Your metabolism is sluggish

Unfortunately, the thinner you are, the lower your metabolic rate tends to be because it takes more energy to run a larger body than a smaller one. So, as you lose weight, your metabolism falls, too.

The easiest and most effective way of speeding up your metabolism is to increase the amount of exercise you do. Be sure to include weight-bearing exercise (like walking or running) because increasing your muscle mass increases your metabolic rate. Eating little and often rather than consuming just a few large meals also may help to boost your metabolism.

You're losing inches instead

Because muscle weighs more than fat, if you're close to your ideal weight and you embark on a program of exercise along with healthy eating, you may find that your body shape changes more than the needle on your scales. You're losing inches and gaining muscle and that may result in a drop in your dress size.

You can measure the change by measuring your waist circumference or by measuring your body fat percentage. As far as your PCOS symptoms are concerned, this type of change is positive because it means that you're losing fat; at the end of the day, fat loss is what helps lessen your PCOS symptoms.

In addition to monitoring weight loss, you may want to keep a record of a few vital statistics, such as waist measurements. When these reduce, you get as much of a positive boost as any weight reduction.

You need to get moving

If you're not active, your calorie requirement to achieve weight loss may need to be less than 1,500. Maintaining a calorie intake as low as this is extremely difficult, and you may also find it hard to get all the nutrients that your body needs at this level of food intake. So, if you're inactive, you may be sticking to the 1,500 but finding that the weight isn't shifting.

You need to get at least 30 minutes a day of some sort of physical activity that gets you slightly out of breath. It doesn't have to be a formal exercise session, and it doesn't have to be all done in one go — three ten-minute sessions work equally well. Exercise that qualifies for this slightly-out-of-breath level includes brisk walking, gardening (especially mowing the lawn with a push mower), swimming at a moderate pace, and bicycling with not too many hills.

Just because you've done your 30 minutes of physical activity for the day, don't think you can rest on your laurels and be a couch potato for the rest of the day. That half-hour of exercise is not a lot when you think it's only half-an-hour out of a 24-hour day, and 8 of those hours are spent in bed! So you need to think about how you can get physically active in your day-to-day life, too. For example, find excuses to run up and down stairs and avoid elevators, or ditch the remote control so that you have to stand up and walk when working the television or stereo. If you work at a desk, get up once in a while to consult with a co-worker face-to-face instead of sending an e-mail to the person down the hall.

You need more sleep

You may think that lying asleep in your bed not doing anything wouldn't help you to burn more calories. But, in fact, the reverse is true. Recent studies show that people who sleep less have a greater increase in body mass and waist circumference over time. Indeed, a lack of sleep has been shown to be associated with an almost twofold increase in obesity levels for both children and adults. Apparently, everyone is getting less and less sleep, so thinking about how much you get is worthwhile because almost a quarter of the adult population is believed to be sleep-deprived.

Symptoms of sleep deprivation include the following:

- ✔ Exhaustion, fatigue, and lack of physical energy
- ✔ Feelings of pessimism, sadness, stress, and anger
- ✔ Memory problems, speech difficulties, and decreased problem-solving abilities

Lack of sleep may lead to obesity because of an increase in appetite that is, in turn, due to the hormonal changes driven by sleep deprivation. Lack of sleep also can make you more stressed, and when you're stressed you produce more of the hormone cortisol, which is believed to lead to a greater tendency for weight to be deposited around your middle, the danger zone.

Lack of sleep is thought to trigger an excessive production of the hormone ghrelin, which causes, among other things, an increase in appetite. Sleep deprivation also is believed to trigger other chronic conditions such as diabetes, high blood pressure, and early signs of aging. However, more research is needed to find out exactly how lack of sleep leads to these conditions and to obesity.

Remembering that to relapse is human

In addition to just getting fed up with the slow or absent rate of weight loss, the other common reason for giving up on a diet completely is just by falling off the wagon and then not being able to motivate yourself back onto it again.

From time to time, you're likely to trip and fall. This lapse doesn't mean that you shouldn't keep trying to reach your goal. Just keep taking more steps forward than backward, and you'll get there!

Remember that feeling too negative about your occasional failures sets you up to give up altogether. If you have a temporary lapse, acknowledge it and try to determine why it happened, but then pick yourself back up and get back on the path to success as soon as you can!

Chapter 6

Let's Get Physical

*N*ext to watching your diet, exercising is the best way to improve your PCOS symptoms and your health in general. Exercise has the added benefit of making you look and feel better about yourself.

So, what are you waiting for? Read on and discover that everyone can get more physically active. You may even start to enjoy it!

Reasons to Get Physical

Researchers keep finding out more and more about the benefits of exercise, from reducing your risk of heart disease and osteoporosis to making you feel happier. Obviously, exercising helps you burn calories, but for those with PCOS, it also reduces insulin resistance, which has the added benefit of improving skin, reducing hair loss, decreasing your risk of diabetes, and increasing fertility.

Talk to your doctor before starting any sort of exercise routine; he is likely to lend enthusiastic support to the idea but may give you some specific advice on how to start and what to do or not do when you make the first move. Although it's not likely that your doctor will completely forbid exercise for medical reasons, he may advise starting slowly with basic exercises rather than jumping right into training for a half-marathon.

To burn calories

Your weight is, essentially, the difference between the energy you take in minus the energy you use up. Exercise is the energy-out part of the equation; the food you eat is the energy-in part. When energy out is greater than energy in, you lose weight.

Your body burns fuel (which is what the energy-out side is all about) in two ways:

- ✔ **Your resting metabolic rate** is the energy you burn just by staying alive. Digesting food, breathing, and thinking all use energy. You burn this energy regardless of whether you're active or just lying on the couch all day. Medical experts call this the *basal metabolic rate*.

- ✔ **Your activity level during the day** is the energy you use by moving around. It includes the energy you use doing your chores, walking to the bus stop, brushing your teeth, and so on, plus any energy you use doing formal exercise.

You don't have much control over your basic metabolic rate, but you have a lot of control over your activity level. Ideally, your exercise regime should include formal exercise — a particular activity that you do for a specific amount of time on a regular schedule — and general activity throughout the day.

Compared to 30 years ago or so, people today get more exercise at the gym and less in their everyday lives. Researchers believe that the daily lack of activity is at least one cause for the rapid rise in obesity levels. Going to the gym is good for fitness and calorie burning, but increasing activity levels goes beyond a few hours a week. Keeping active all day helps you burn calories better than a short, sharp burst of activity followed by little else.

Starting a formal exercise program

So, how much formal exercise should you do on a regular basis?

- ✔ The Centers for Disease Control and Prevention recommends 150 minutes of moderate-intensity physical activity like brisk walking per week. This level of activity may help offset that gradual weight gain that creeps up on women over time.

- ✔ Do muscle-strengthening activities two or more days per week, working all the major muscle groups, including the legs, hips, back, abdomen, chest, shoulders, and arms.

Facts and figures on exercise and weight loss

Research done by the National Weight Control Registry (a registry of around 4,000 people who have successfully maintained a minimum 30-pound weight loss for at least one year) has shown that

✔ Around 90 percent of people used both diet and physical activity to lose weight. Only 9 percent used diet alone, and only 1 percent managed to lose weight through exercise alone. What this means is that the combination of physical activity and watching your calorie intake is more effective for weight loss — and maintenance of weight loss — than cutting calorie intake alone.

✔ Participating in a high level of physical activity predicted successful weight-loss maintenance. In fact, participants did 60 to 90 minutes of moderately intense physical activity a day (equivalent to brisk walking, cycling, or jogging at a rate of around 250 to 350 calories per hour), amounting to an extra calorie expenditure of around 2,500 calories per week.

✔ Walking was the most popular form of physical activity, but most people also participated in other exercise sessions, too. In fact, only 28 percent used walking alone as their exercise, while about 50 percent combined walking with another form of planned physical activity, such as aerobics classes, cycling, or swimming.

✔ Participants who wore pedometers to measure how much they walked in a day found they walked 5½ to 6 miles per day, or 11,000 to 12,000 steps.

Exercise needs to be something sustained that gets your heart rate up, such as brisk walking, digging a garden, mowing the lawn (with a push mower), swimming, or cycling. For example, if you do 30 to 35 minutes of moderately intense exercise (such as jogging or cycling), you burn around an extra 300 calories a day. Exercising five days a week will give you a 1,500-calorie-per-week deficit, which will rid you of almost half a pound a week without changing your diet at all.

Going for general activity

If you engage in some type of formal exercise regime, great. But what about working on your general level of activity for the rest of the day?

Here are some ideas on how you can get more active throughout the day:

✔ **Take the stairs rather than the elevator.**

✔ **Park at the far end of the parking lot.** Let other people take the parking spaces close to the door.

✔ **Hide the remote control.** This way, you have to physically get up and walk to the TV to change channels — and while you're up, take a quick jog around the room!

✔ **Exercise while watching TV.** For example, you can use a *resistance band* (a stretchy rubber tube with handles on both ends) to give your muscles some resistance training.

✔ **Burn extra calories doing household chores.** Put some elbow grease into activities like polishing, vacuuming, and stretching for cobwebs. Don't think of it as a chore — think of it as a mini-workout!

✔ **Turn into a fidgeter.** Fidgeters are people who just can't keep still; they're always jiggling their legs or wriggling around in their seats. Fidgeting burns calories, so fidgeters tend to weigh less than people who sit perfectly still, although they may annoy the people who have to sit next to them!

Looking at how many calories you need to burn

To lose a pound of body weight, you need to take in around 3,500 calories less than you expend. This equation works in reverse too; to gain a pound, you need to eat an extra 3,500 calories.

For this reason, exercise alone is unlikely to burn enough calories to add up to a lot of weight loss, unless you're working out intensely every day. Don't sweat it — we're not suggesting high-intensity workouts, which are impractical for most people and not necessary to maintain health. Table 6-1 gives you an idea of how many calories different activities use. The figures listed are for a woman weighing 140 pounds performing the activity for 30 minutes.

You burn more calories if you're heavier to start with because it takes more work for you to move your body around.

Table 6-1   Energy Costs of Various Activities

Activity	*Energy Cost (Calories per 30 Minutes)*
Leisurely walking	80
Weight lifting	101
General housework	118

Activity	Energy Cost (Calories per 30 Minutes)
General gardening	151
Golf (carrying clubs)	185
Low-impact aerobics	185
Mowing the lawn with a push mower	185
Very brisk walking	200
Shoveling snow by hand	202
High-impact aerobics	235
Rowing machine, moderate	235
Stationary cycle machine	235
Tennis	235
Running (5 mph)	267
Bicycling (12–14 mph)	269
Boxing/sparring	302
Jumping rope	336

To pump up your metabolism

The energy you use just by existing on planet Earth accounts for the biggest chunk of your overall calorie expenditure. When you exercise, you not only burn calories during the exercise but also boost your basal metabolism a notch for an hour or so after working out, an added benefit of exercise that costs nothing extra!

Muscle is much more metabolically active than fat. So, losing fat and building more muscle increases your basal metabolism rate, so you burn more calories even when you're sleeping.

Muscle is heavier than fat, so you can actually lose a lot of your body fat but not register any weight loss on the scales. You may, however, notice the difference in your clothing size and how toned you look.

As you get older, you tend to lose muscle mass as a natural conse-
quence of aging, especially from the upper body. Muscle turns to
fat and congregates around your waist, just where you don't want
it! But you can fight back: Exercising regularly and working your
upper body with a few weights can offset that muscle loss. (See the
"Resistance work" section later in this chapter.)

Losing weight, especially if you lose rapidly, results in muscle
tissue loss as well as fat loss. Your scales may register a weight
loss, but it's not all good news! If you don't exercise while losing
weight, you lose muscle with fat, which can lower your metabolic
rate. If you subsequently put some weight back on, it goes back
on as fat and then if you lose this again by dieting and not exercising, you lower your muscle mass and metabolic rate even more,
making it harder to avoid further weight gain. No wonder losing
and regaining weight too often ends up as a yo-yo syndrome.

Invest in some body fat measuring scales so that you can keep an
eye on what's happening to your body fat level as you lose weight.
(See Chapter 5 for more details on how to interpret these scales.)

Being active protects from a variety of cancers

Maintaining a healthy body weight and staying active may reduce your cancer risk.
Inactivity increases your risk of colon and breast cancer; being very active may
halve your risk of colon cancer. Physical activity protects against breast cancer
in women both before and after menopause, but scientists see the greatest risk
reductions in women who are active before menopause. As with bowel cancer,
physical activity probably reduces breast cancer risk by lowering levels of insulin,
hormones, and growth factors. Some evidence exists that physical activity can
alter estrogen metabolism to produce weaker versions of this hormone, reducing
the cancer-promoting effect that estrogen can have on the body.

Inactivity also may be linked to cancers of the uterus and lung. A recent analysis of
several studies found that high physical activity reduced the risk of lung cancer by
about 30 percent. Being active may reduce lung cancer risk by improving the lung's
efficiency. This may reduce the time that cancer-causing chemicals spend in the
lung, as well as lowering their concentration.

Being overweight or obese can greatly increase your risk of cancer, and if you have
PCOS you're more likely to carry some extra weight. To reduce your cancer risk, get
30 minutes of moderate physical activity five times a week.

To look great

Having PCOS may make you feel unattractive, but exercise can help. By exercising, you get

- **A healthy glow to your skin.**

- **More definition and sculpturing of the body as your muscles develop, even if you don't lose weight:** Women don't tend to build up bulk in their muscles as men do, but their muscles definitely become more defined.

- **More of a defined waist as your waist circumference decreases, which is a great PCOS symptom-reducer:** Clothes hang much better on your more sculptured frame.

- **Improved mood, confidence, and feelings of well-being:** When you feel good inside, you look better on the outside!

To increase your happiness factor

After about ten minutes of the kind of exercise that gets you slightly out of breath, the body starts to produce hormones called *endorphins,* which give you a natural high and happy feeling. In fact, you typically feel more energized after you've exercised than before (unless, of course, you've overdone it). Physical activity can help overcome depression, sometimes a side effect of PCOS.

To reduce the symptoms of PCOS

Being physically active can help reduce most PCOS symptoms, mainly because exercise reduces insulin resistance. (See Chapter 3 for more on insulin resistance.)

Most insulin resistance occurs mainly in muscle tissue. Because muscle tissue can't properly utilize insulin, more insulin must be pumped out by the pancreas before it can start to have an effect. Being physically inactive further aggravates insulin resistance. So, by incorporating plenty of physical activity, you get these benefits:

- You make your body more receptive to the effects of insulin, so less insulin is produced.

- You increase the rate at which glucose gets used up (to help generate energy for the muscles). This means that less insulin is needed to bring down blood sugar levels.

- Lowered insulin levels lead to a more regular menstrual cycle and, thus, to better fertility. (See Chapter 10 for more about PCOS and the menstrual cycle.)

✔ PCOS symptoms such as acne and hirsutism decrease.

✔ PCOS increases your risk of developing type 2 diabetes. Increasing your exercise level (even if you don't actually lose weight) can lower your risk.

Accumulating fat around the waist is a known side effect of PCOS. Abdominal fat increases your risk of developing insulin resistance and all the PCOS symptoms that go with it. Research shows that exercise may be especially helpful in reducing the size of fat cells around the waistline — more so than diet alone. When obese women were placed on a regimen of calorie cutting alone or diet plus exercise, those who exercised showed a reduction in the size of fat cells around the abdomen; women who only dieted showed no such change. However, both groups trimmed about the same amount of fat cells from the hip area. Exercise targeted the waist — the most dangerous place to be carrying fat.

To reap other health rewards

Here are some other positive health effects of exercise:

✔ It reduces the risk of osteoporosis.

✔ It raises the level of "good" cholesterol (HDL) in the blood, helping to protect you from heart disease.

✔ It generally reduces the risk of developing heart disease and strokes.

✔ It lowers blood pressure.

✔ It makes you feel less tired and lethargic and may improve sleep.

✔ It decreases constipation.

✔ It helps you look and feel younger and may also help you live longer.

✔ It reduces stress and anxiety levels.

Ground Rules before You Start

Don't just jump into a new exercise regimen without doing some planning and research. Lack of planning and not thinking realistically about your goals are part of the reason lifestyle changes often don't stick.

Getting the green light from your doctor

If you have a medical condition, such as PCOS and are overweight, tell your doctor whenever you plan to join any classes or engage in more taxing exercise. She may want to check your heart and lungs. If you have joint problems or are obese, your doctor may suggest avoiding some exercises at first.

Overcoming common barriers

Unfortunately, 50 percent of people who start on an exercise program drop out within six months, particularly if they're overweight. But if you can keep up an exercise routine beyond six months, you'll have established a routine that's more likely to stick for the long term.

Table 6-2 lists common barriers (and excuses!) to exercise and how to overcome them.

Table 6-2	Barriers to Physical Activity and How to Overcome Them
Common Barrier	**Possible Solution**
Lack of time	You can always make time, even if it's only 20 minutes a day. Build exercise into your daily routines and possibly save money at the same time by walking or bicycling to the store instead of driving. Park farther away from the store if you drive — every step counts!
Lack of money	Exercise is free. Taking a brisk walk or jog costs nothing, but it pays big dividends!
Lack of support	Starting an exercise program is more fun with friends. Exercise with people you know — even your kids! — or start off with a few sessions with a personal trainer.
Accessibility	You don't need to be within easy reach of a gym or have access to a car. You can work out in your own living room with an exercise DVD. Invest in an exercise trampoline, which can be turned on its side to take up very little space when not in use. Plus, the big outdoors is never more than a few steps away.

(continued)

Table 6-2 *(continued)*

Previous negative experience	You may still be smarting from the embarrassment of being picked last in gym class. Or you may have recently joined an exercise class and felt humiliated. But you can rise above that! Find other people to go with you — there's safety in numbers!
Feeling too embarrassed because of appearance	In exercise class, most people are too worried about how *they* look to worry about how *you* look. Buy some exercise clothing that makes you feel good, or go with a friend for added confidence. If you feel really embarrassed by your appearance, start off at home and build up to more public exercise when you feel more comfortable.
Feeling too unfit	Everyone starts somewhere, however unfit they are. If you stick with it, you'll be pleasantly surprised by how quickly you notice a change in your fitness level, mood, and appearance. Start with ten minutes and build up, starting with yoga, Pilates, or other stretching classes to get your body used to moving before turning up the heat.

Customizing your workout

Keep in mind the following when choosing an exercise:

✔ **Heed your health professional's advice.** If he suggests avoiding certain exercises, keep these restrictions in mind.

✔ **Think realistically about how much time you can devote to working out.** Don't sabotage your success by trying to do too much too fast.

✔ **Plan exercise around your daily routine, such as walking rather than taking the car.** This helps you stay active throughout the day and increases the odds that you'll stick with it. After all, if you walked to the store, you have to walk home!

✔ **Include your kids in your exercise regime.** Keeping your kids active physically has health benefits for them, too. Go swimming or take long walks as a family for bonding time as well as exercise.

✔ **If competitive sports are your thing, join an organized team of whatever appeals to you.** Even golf is an exercise — just leave the cart at the club!

✔ **If you like company while you exercise, choose exercise classes or group activities with friends or family.**

✔ **You can exercise for free or pay for classes at a gym.** You may want to mix and match — go to class twice a week and do an exercise DVD at home in between.

✔ **Combine exercise and boost your social life at the same time.** Go dancing and meet some new people. Many colleges or adult education centers offer dance classes for nominal fees.

✔ **Learn self-defense and get fit at the same time by joining a martial arts class, such as Tae Kwan Do or kick boxing.** These activities will definitely raise your heart rate!

✔ **If motivation is an issue, consider investing in a personal trainer.** Knowing you've spent the money may motivate you to keep going back.

You're much more likely to keep up regular physical activity if you enjoy it and it fits into your daily life.

Not All Exercise Is the Same

To get the full benefit of being active and reduce your PCOS symptoms, you need a mixture of three different types of exercise:

✔ **Aerobic exercise:** Do aerobic exercise every day if possible, but at least for five days of the week and for a minimum of 30 minutes per day. You can do your aerobic exercise in 10-minute increments throughout the day, if you prefer — you don't have to do all 30 minutes at once.

✔ **Resistance training:** Do resistance exercises two to three times a week, but leave a day between each session if you can, or exercise a different set of muscles if you're training on consecutive days.

✔ **Flexibility:** Do some flexibility exercises as part of your stretching after each aerobic workout. If you find it relaxing, take a Pilates, T'ai Chi, or similar class (see the "Maintaining flexibility" section, later); you can do one of these once a week or every day if you prefer.

Each of these types of exercise has different effects and benefits. Ideally, you need a combination of all three types of exercise throughout the week.

Aerobic exercise

One definition of *aerobic exercise* is "sustained exercise that uses large muscle groups and places demands on the cardiovascular system." In other words, the type of exercise that gets your heart pumping and leaves you a bit out of breath.

If you have PCOS, aerobic exercise has the following benefits:

✔ It improves the condition of your heart and lungs.

✔ It reduces insulin levels and insulin resistance.

✔ It lowers blood sugar levels.

✔ It helps lower blood pressure.

✔ It lifts your mood.

✔ It speeds up your metabolism and makes you burn more calories, both during and after exercise.

Aerobic exercise explained

Any exercise that increases your breathing and heart rate and warms you up can be called aerobic, including walking (if done briskly enough), jogging, running, digging in the garden, and dancing.

Experts recommend that you do at least 30 minutes of some sort of aerobic activity five times a week. If you haven't done any aerobic exercise for a while, you may need to start slowly and visit your doctor before you start.

 If finding the time to do a solid half-hour of aerobic exercise is difficult, doing it in ten-minute increments is fine. Walking briskly to the bus stop, taking another brisk walk at lunchtime, mowing your lawn, or pushing the vacuum cleaner around the house briskly for ten minutes all add up.

Walking as a form of aerobic activity

Walking is cheap, easy, and good for you. If you have PCOS and you're carrying around some extra weight, walking is an ideal exercise that doesn't put too much stress on your joints. Plus, walking is the exercise people are most likely to continue as they get older.

Fit yourself with a pedometer

Pedometers are little gadgets that fit to your waist band and measure how many steps you take.

Many people overestimate their activity levels. Pedometers can give you a more accurate picture of how active you are. You may be shocked to find out how few steps you take in a typical day. Taking a minimum of 10,000 steps per day helps improve health.

Pedometers can be a great motivational tool. Keeping a log of your steps may help motivate you to keep it up. Pedometers also can translate steps into actual distance and calories burned. Read the instructions that come with the pedometer so you learn how to wear the pedometer properly to get an accurate reading.

Use the first week with your pedometer to establish a base line for future comparison — go about your normal routine while wearing your pedometer without changing your activity pattern. When you know your current activity level, adjust it upward if possible. Set a goal that you can reach (for example, an additional 200 steps per day). When you reach that goal, set a new goal for yourself.

A regular walking program can result in some of the following benefits:

- ✔ Lowered resting heart rate (which is a sign of general fitness)
- ✔ Reduced blood pressure
- ✔ The expending of calories
- ✔ Reduced stress levels
- ✔ Increased muscle tone
- ✔ Weight loss
- ✔ Reduced risk of heart attack or stroke

Walking is a fantastic way to start introducing some exercise into your life, because you can start really slowly. It doesn't require a lot of equipment or a special place to do it. Plus, you can keep up your exercise program even when you're traveling.

Experts recommend that you work up to about 45 minutes three to four times per week. That should be the goal, not something you do right away. Shorter distances and less time are the watchwords when starting out.

Getting started on your walking program

Here are some ground rules before you start a walking program:

✔ Wear a good pair of shoes; sturdy heel support is imperative.

✔ Dress appropriately for the time of year. Wear layers so you can shed them if you get too warm.

✔ Walk in daylight or well-lit areas at night. Wear reflective clothes if you do walk at night.

✔ Walk with someone else, if possible. Dogs make great walking companions.

✔ Don't wear headphones. They can prevent you from hearing a car or other forms of danger.

Resistance work

Resistance training includes weight training, weight-machine use, and resistance-band workouts.

Technically, *resistance training* literally means working against a weight, force, or gravity.

Resistance training has the following benefits:

✔ It increases your strength, muscular endurance, and muscle size.

✔ It helps boost metabolic rate and, thus, fat-burning capacity. Muscle tissue is estimated to be up to 70 times more metabolically active than fat — really important if you have PCOS!

✔ It helps reduce insulin resistance, which is vital to reduce PCOS symptoms.

✔ It may help lower blood pressure, which has a tendency to be higher in PCOS.

✔ It helps offset osteoporosis, because bones are strengthened by bearing weight and by the pull of active muscles.

✔ It helps offset lower-back pain and other muscular problems.

✔ It improves your balance and stability.

✔ It keeps your muscles primed and ready for action. With muscle strength and functionality, it tends to be a case of "use it or lose it."

Research indicates that virtually all the benefits of resistance training are likely to be obtained in two 15- to 20-minute training sessions per week.

Practical aspects of resisting

Sensible resistance training involves precise, controlled movements for each major muscle group and doesn't require the use of very heavy weights.

You can incorporate this kind of exercise into your exercise routine in several ways:

✔ **Using your own body weight such as doing bent-knee sit-ups or abdominal curls, push-ups, and chin-ups:** Using your own body weight is convenient and free. However, when you're strong enough to cope with your own body weight, you need to add devices such as resistance bands or free weights.

✔ **Using resistance bands:** These bands are portable and can be adapted to most workouts. For example, to work the biceps, you step on the band, hold the other end in your fist, and curl up and down. Unlike free weights, the bands provide continuous resistance throughout a movement. However, bands don't exert as much force on the muscle as a free weight, which means they may be better suited for gentle shaping and toning.

✔ **Using free weights, such as dumbbells or barbells:** Free weights can be used to target every muscle in the body. Generally, you need a gym membership or a set of weights at home. However, beginners can use everyday household items for dumbbells, such as a couple of soup cans. Just don't drop them on your foot!

✔ **Using weight machines:** Weight machines have adjustable seats with handles attached to either weights or hydraulics. Weight machines are helpful for beginners because they guide the movement and ensure good form. However, you can't always adjust a weight machine to get the perfect fit for your body size and shape.

Most fitness experts suggest that you use weights that you can lift 8 to 12 times. You may then repeat this whole set two to three times.

Wait 24 to 48 hours between resistance-training sessions for a particular set of muscles. However, you can work on a different set of muscles within that time.

Pumping iron slows middle-age spread

Research has shown that a twice-weekly strength-training regimen slows the accumulation of so-called middle-age spread. And because women with PCOS often develop middle-age spread before the fact, it's particularly useful for them!

Researchers divided a group of overweight or obese women between ages 25 and 44 into two groups. One group was given diet advice and told to exercise moderately to vigorously for 30 minutes on most days of the week (but no checks were made on whether they carried through any of the advice). The other group was given supervised robust resistance training by trained instructors. Both groups were told to keep their weight steady.

The body fat was measured using a CAT scan at base line and then after two years.

After the two-year period, both groups had not changed their body weight, but *visceral fat* (the fat around the middle) had increased by 20 percent in the group told to exercise and given dietary advice, whereas those who were trained to pump iron gained only 6 percent visceral fat. Weight training decreased middle-age spread!

If done incorrectly, weight training can end up doing you more harm than good, so if you're totally new to this type of exercise, ask a professional for weight-lifting advice.

Check out *Weight Training For Dummies,* 3rd Edition, by Liz Neporent, Suzanne Schlosberg, and Shirley J. Archer (Wiley), for more information on weight training.

Maintaining flexibility

Being supple and flexible improves your posture and balance and allows you to maintain full movements throughout your body. Although this isn't essential to helping with PCOS symptoms, being flexible is part of the whole getting-fit package that helps you look better and feel better about yourself.

Stretching

To maintain suppleness and prevent muscles and joints from stiffening up, always stretch your muscles before and after an exercise session, whether you're doing resistance training, aerobic training, or both.

Here are some advantages of stretching:

✔ It enhances physical fitness.

✔ It can increase mental and physical relaxation.

✔ It can help reduce the risk of injury to joints, muscles, and tendons.

✔ It helps prevent or reduce muscular soreness.

✔ It helps to increase suppleness by stimulating the production of chemicals that lubricate joints.

✔ It may even help to reduce the severity of painful menstruation.

 Never over-force yourself into a stretch or bounce yourself into it; just let your body relax into the stretch, or you may injure yourself. Again, get advice from a qualified fitness instructor or a good DVD (or check out *Stretching For Dummies*, by LaReine Chabut with Madeleine Lewis [Wiley]). If you have any injuries, or muscle or joint problems, seek professional help before starting.

Flexibility exercise

Like muscle use, putting the various joints of your body through their paces and reminding them of the movements they should be able to do helps prevent you from becoming stiff. Lots of classes are offered that build in a high degree of flexibility, including

✔ **Yoga:** A system of exercises aimed at helping you control your body and mind, as well as improving your breathing and focusing the alignment of your body

✔ **Pilates:** A form of exercise that aims to help develop body awareness, improve posture and alignment, and increase flexibility and ease of movement

✔ **T'ai Chi:** Combines movement, meditation, and breath regulation with the aim of enhancing the flow of vital energy in the body, improving blood circulation, and enhancing immune functions

Such classes also help to improve your posture, balance breath control, and reduce symptoms of stress. If you have PCOS, they're a very gentle way to start exercising and still give you a bit of a workout without getting worn out and discouraged. When you find exercise a bit easier and even fun, add more strenuous exercises to have more effect on PCOS symptoms.

Exercise in pregnancy

Here are some general guidelines about exercise during pregnancy. This advice applies to all women, regardless of whether they have PCOS:

- ✔ If you were physically active before getting pregnant, continuing to exercise is fine, as long as the exercise is moderately intensive and doesn't go beyond about 30 to 40 minutes. Running marathons is probably out.

- ✔ Avoid exercise that involves long durations of intense training.

- ✔ Exercising aerobically three to four times per week is probably the limit during pregnancy, for no more than 30 to 40 minutes at a time.

- ✔ Non-weight-bearing exercise, such as gentle cycling or swimming, is particularly recommended (although in late pregnancy you may want to stick to a stationary bike, because you're less likely to fall).

- ✔ In the third trimester, avoid any exercises that involve lying flat on your back.

As soon as you know you're pregnant, check with your doctor about whether exercising is okay. As someone with PCOS, you may have had problems with miscarriage in the past. Ask your medical practitioner about what exercises you can do and what you should avoid.

Eating for Exercise

Unless you're training to be an elite athlete, you don't have to worry too much about what you eat to get the best out of your physical activity sessions. Just follow the dietary advice throughout this book to help you with your PCOS. If you're following a low-GI, balanced diet and following the guidelines in Chapter 4, you're doing well.

Here are some basic guidelines that can help you maximize the benefits of physical activity while eating a balanced diet suitable for PCOS:

- ✔ Eat a wide variety of foods to ensure that you have all the nutrients your body needs to function at its peak.

- ✔ If you drink alcohol, do so in moderation, but avoid drinking before or immediately after exercise.

> ✔ Make sure that you're well hydrated both before and after you exercise.
>
> ✔ If you sweat during exercise, remember to drink extra water to compensate for the fluid lost in sweat.
>
> ✔ Eat plenty of low-GI carbs. Because the energy release from low- to medium-GI foods is more sustained, this type of food may help you to exercise more efficiently without running out of steam. (See Chapter 4 for more on eating a low-GI diet.)
>
> ✔ Eat at least five portions of fruits or vegetables every day.
>
> ✔ Eat less fat and replace saturated fats with unsaturated ones.
>
> ✔ Eat moderate amounts of protein.
>
> ✔ Eat two portions of fish a week, one of which should be oily.
>
> ✔ Don't exercise on a full stomach or after a big meal.
>
> ✔ If you exercise every day, eat smaller main meals with snacks in between to keep up your energy levels.

Workout fuel

What you eat before exercise can make the difference between an energetic (perhaps even peppy) workout and a tired, looking-at-your-watch-every-five-minutes workout. Follow these basic guidelines for fueling your workouts.

Early-morning workouts

If you like morning workouts (before your body has a chance to protest), nibble on something to avoid feeling dizzy and hungry. Allow enough time for your food to digest to avoid cramping or, worse, nausea. Try the following:

> ✔ If you're exercising within an hour after you wake up, eat 200 to 300 calories before your workout.
>
> ✔ Keep fat intake low, because fat can hang around in the stomach for a while, waiting to be digested and making you feel uncomfortable when you work out.

Good food choices for early-morning workouts include whole-grain cereals, raisins, bananas, or a blended fruit and milk-based drink. Or try a couple slices of whole-grain bread with mashed-up banana and a little peanut butter.

Lunchtime workouts

By lunchtime, breakfast is probably a faint memory. In order to avoid hunger pangs and fatigue during your lunchtime workout, have a low-GI, low-fat, carbohydrate-rich snack one or two hours before your workout. Good choices include a milkshake, whole-grain crackers with peanut butter or hummus, yogurt, fruit (fresh or dried), or a small bowl of a low-GI cereal. Also, make sure that you eat a balanced meal after your workout.

After-work workouts

The workday's done, you're on the way to the gym, and you're *hungry*. Does your steering wheel mysteriously turn your car in the direction of the nearest fast-food restaurant? That's because lunch was a long time ago and your body is out of fuel. You need to follow the same advice given for those who work out at lunch: Have a low-GI, low-fat, carbohydrate-rich snack one or two hours before your workout. And eat a balanced meal afterward.

After the workout

When you're finished exercising, you need to replace some of those calories you burned; if you've worked out intensely, your glycogen reserves are likely to be low and need replacing.

Glycogen is your body's easily accessible source of fuel, which gets converted rapidly to glucose during activity. Failing to replace your glycogen reserves (which are stored in the liver and muscles) means that you have very little energy reserves left for the next time you need to do anything even slightly energetic.

To replace your glycogen reserves, ensure that your after-workout meal is a good source of carbs. Having some protein with those carbs may further enhance the body's ability to restock glycogen.

Don't wait too long after exercise before you grab yourself a meal or a snack, otherwise you may find yourself completely out of energy.

Chapter 7

Taking Medications

. . . .

In This Chapter

▶ Going the drug route to treat PCOS

▶ Reducing insulin resistance

▶ Controlling your blood glucose levels

▶ Getting your periods on schedule

▶ Minimizing acne and hairiness

▶ Putting a halt to endometrial buildup

▶ Losing weight

. . . .

*P*COS has the dubious distinction of being the most common hormonal disorder in women of reproductive age. Despite this, there is no cure for the disorder, and most treatments are aimed at improving the symptoms. However, certain medications can definitely help treat the symptoms, and some medications attempt to treat the underlying cause of PCOS: insulin resistance. In this chapter, we look at the drugs available and talk about the pros and cons of using them.

Following the Current Medical Approach

The typical American approach to medical issues is to take a pill in the hopes that the condition will go away. Although some medications may help the symptoms of PCOS fade into the background, they won't cure the disorder.

That doesn't mean that the medications aren't worth taking, though. Reducing the symptoms — particularly major symptoms like insulin resistance — can start a domino effect that improves other symptoms as well. Some of the drugs used to treat PCOS are used *off-label* — meaning that they were tested and approved in clinical trials for other medical uses. (See the sidebar "What does *off-label* mean?" for more about off-label drug use.)

Table 7-1 lists some of the common symptoms of PCOS and which drugs may be prescribed for them. The following sections go into more detail.

Table 7-1 PCOS Symptoms and Treatments

Symptom	Treatment
High cholesterol levels	Statins
Insulin resistance, reducing blood glucose levels	Metformin, thiazolidinediones, acarbose
Poor development of the *endometrium* (the lining of the uterus)	Natural or synthetic progestogens/progesterones
Irregular periods	Combination estrogen/progestin contraceptive methods, including pills, patches, or rings
Lack of ovulation, infertility	Clomid and chorionic gonadotrophin, follicle-stimulating hormone (FSH)
Depression	Anti-depressive agents such as selective serotonin reuptake inhibitors (SSRIs)
Hirsutism (excessive hair growth) and acne	Anti-androgens, aladactone (anti-testosterone diuretics), topical anti-hirsutism cream, statins
Obesity	Orlistat, sibutramine, rimonabant

Taking prescribed medication is not an easy way out to escape the hard work of exercising or dieting. Drugs tend to have side effects and can interact negatively with each other. Starting with diet and exercise can reduce your reliance on medications.

What does *off-label* mean?

Drugs used *off-label* have undergone testing to prove their safety and effectiveness for certain disorders, but their effectiveness for the condition being treated off-label has not been tested in a clinical trial and presented to the Food and Drug Administration (FDA). That doesn't mean they won't work — almost all these medications and devices have been used by physicians in studies that were not sponsored by the drug companies. These results have been verified and published in peer-reviewed journals and are, thus, valid uses even if they aren't FDA approved and not on the label.

In the case of PCOS, drugs such as anti-diabetic medications and birth control pills are used off-label to treat PCOS. Anti-diabetics were tested for effectiveness in lowering blood glucose, but because insulin resistance is part of both type 2 diabetes and PCOS, the same drug works for both. With birth control pills, the pills were designed and tested for their effectiveness in preventing pregnancy, not decreasing the side effects of PCOS, but the hormones they contain can decrease the amount of circulating *androgens* (male hormones), which helps PCOS.

Treating Insulin Resistance

Several classes of drugs are used to treat insulin resistance, one of the prime causes of the cascade of symptoms that can affect women with PCOS. All have different actions and side effects.

Measuring metformin

Metformin (sold as Glucophage) belongs to a class of medications called biguanides. Biguanides reduce the amount of glucose produced by the liver and improve the uptake of glucose into the cells. Because of these actions, metformin was first used to treat type 2 diabetes, previously known as adult-onset diabetes.

Because metformin improves the body's response to insulin, allowing it to function more effectively, the drug is used off-label to treat PCOS as well as type 2 diabetes. Taking metformin may keep you from developing type 2 diabetes (which is associated with insulin resistance) down the road.

Metformin is useful for treating PCOS because it helps with the following:

- ✔ Reducing insulin resistance
- ✔ Reducing insulin production
- ✔ Losing weight
- ✔ Reducing androgen levels
- ✔ Restoring normal blood fat levels
- ✔ Reducing the high long-term risk of heart disease in PCOS
- ✔ Improving regularity of menstrual cycles
- ✔ Improving fertility

Doctors and PCOS medical experts are split on how effective metformin is in the treatment of PCOS. Although metformin does improve the symptoms of PCOS, some studies show that diet and exercise, when adhered to, are as effective in lowering androgen levels and regulating menstrual periods.

Metformin can give rise to an assortment of unpleasant gastrointestinal effects in between 5 percent and 20 percent of people, including

- ✔ Abdominal discomfort
- ✔ Bloating
- ✔ Diarrhea
- ✔ Gas
- ✔ Loss of appetite
- ✔ Nausea
- ✔ Vomiting

Perhaps more seriously, metformin also can lead to poor vitamin B12 absorption in 10 percent to 30 percent of cases, which can lead to anemia from B12 deficiency.

Metformin also can increase your homocysteine levels. Homocysteines are *amino acids,* the building blocks of protein, found in the blood. High levels of homocysteines increases your risk of developing heart disease such as *atherosclerosis,* a buildup of plaque in the arteries that can lead to heart attack or stroke.

Rarely, a serious condition known as *lactic acidosis* can occur in people taking metformin. Lactic acidosis develops when muscles release lactic acid during exercise. Lactic acid builds up in the blood when the liver can't convert it to glucose quickly enough. This buildup of acid in the blood can lead to coma or, in 35 percent to 50 percent of cases, death. Women most at risk of developing lactic acidosis are those with liver or kidney disease, alcohol abusers, and those who are dehydrated or who have infections.

On the positive side, metformin does not cause low blood sugar or weight gain, common side effects of other drugs used to lower insulin levels.

Metformin is normally taken two to three times a day, although a once-a-day extended-release form is available. The extended-release form may cause fewer gastrointestinal symptoms.

Taking thiazolidinediones

Other insulin-sensitizing medications include the thiazolidinediones such as rosiglitazone (sold as Avandia; see the nearby sidebar, "The FDA's major move on Avandia") and pioglitazone (sold as Actos). Thiazolidinediones enhance insulin sensitivity by attaching to insulin receptor cells throughout the body, which makes them more receptive to insulin. These drugs are sometimes used in conjunction with metformin.

Like metformin, thiazolidinediones come with a formidable list of side effects, which can differ depending on the particular drug. Side effects of rosiglitazones include the following:

- ✔ Backache
- ✔ Diarrhea
- ✔ *Edema* (fluid retention)
- ✔ Headache
- ✔ *Hypoglycemia* (low blood glucose levels)
- ✔ Weight gain

More serious side effects include worsening heart failure from edema and an increased risk of chest pain and heart attack. Taking rosiglitazones for four to six years also can increase your risk of bone fractures. These drugs tend to be used more for thin PCOS sufferers who don't tolerate metformin very well.

The FDA's major move on Avandia

In 2010, the FDA, in conjunction with drug-regulating agencies throughout Europe, put severe limits on the availability of Avandia for treatment of type 2 diabetes. Although European agencies banned the drug altogether, the FDA has restricted its use to people whose doctors can prove that they've tried other drugs to lower blood glucose levels and that patients have been told of the potentially serious heart effects of Avandia.

Rezulin, a similar drug in the same class, was taken off the market in 1999 because it caused liver damage in some cases. Actos, the last drug in this class on the market, appears to affect different genes than the other two drugs and doesn't have the same side effects.

If you take Avandia for PCOS or as an anti-diabetic, talk with your doctor about possible alternatives.

Picking up pioglitazones

Actos, another drug approved to treat type 2 diabetes and used off-label to treat PCOS in some cases, also increases your body's sensitivity to insulin. Actos does have side effects, including the following:

- ✔ Headache
- ✔ Muscle aches
- ✔ Runny nose or other cold symptoms
- ✔ Sore throat

More serious side effects include the following:

- ✔ Worsening congestive heart failure, which causes fluid retention and swelling, shortness of breath, frequent dry cough, and difficulty sleeping unless your head is elevated

- ✔ Liver disease, signs of which include nausea, yellowish tinge to your skin or the whites of your eyes, dark urine, pale stools, abdominal pain, or fatigue

- ✔ Vision changes, including blurred vision or vision loss

- ✔ Hypoglycemia, which causes shakiness, weakness, sweating, headache, difficulty concentrating, and sometimes even coma

Actos also may increase your chances of developing bladder cancer. Clinical trials to assess the drug for this potential effect are currently underway.

Reducing Blood Glucose Levels

Biguanides and other insulin-sensitizing medications can be used to treat type 2 diabetes as well as PCOS, because that's what they're primarily designed and tested for. A number of other drugs also can be used to lower blood glucose levels if you have type 2 diabetes.

Acarbose

Acarbose, sold in the United States as Precose, is a drug that stops carbohydrates from being broken down into glucose in the gut by inhibiting the action of certain enzymes. Unless carbs are broken down to their simple-sugar state, they can't be absorbed into the bloodstream. The most common simple sugar broken down from carbohydrates is glucose. After it's absorbed into the bloodstream, glucose requires insulin in order for the cells to use or store it.

Acarbose can cause annoying digestive side effects (mostly gas), which are due to bacterial fermentation of undigested carbs sloshing around in the gut.

A recent study shows that treatment with acarbose in women with PCOS leads to reduced acne, better insulin response to a glucose load, and more normal androgen levels.

Sitagliptin

Sitagliptin (sold as Januvia) increases your insulin output and decreases the amount of glucose your liver produces. Januvia is less likely to cause low blood glucose level than other oral anti-diabetic medications. In rare cases, Januvia has caused inflammation of the pancreas. Abdominal pain, nausea, vomiting, and appetite loss may occur if you have pancreatitis.

More common side effects include the following:

- Headache
- Diarrhea
- Constipation
- Nausea

Regulating Periods

Birth control pills usually are recommended to women with PCOS who don't want to become pregnant in order to regulate their menstrual cycles and to possibly improve some of the PCOS-related symptoms. In women with PCOS who experience absent periods, the synthetic progestins in birth control pills also help protect their uterine lining from changes that may eventually lead to endometrial cancer.

Birth control pills and other contraceptives such as the vaginal ring or skin patch fall into one of several different categories. These birth control methods can contain

- ✔ Synthetic estrogen in the form of ethinyl estradiol and progestin available in several types taken in equal amounts all month, called *monophasic pills*

- ✔ Synthetic estrogen and progestin taken in varying amounts during the month, called *biphasicpills* or *triphasic pills*

- ✔ Progestin only

The progestins used in birth control pills include levonorgestrel, norethindrone acetate, desogestrel, norgestimate, norethindrone, norgestrel, ethynodiol diacetate, and drospirenone.

Birth control pills regulate your menstrual cycles by building up your uterine lining with ethinyl estradiol and progestins for three weeks. At the end of three weeks, you have a withdrawal bleed, an effect caused by the withdrawal of progesterone. This is not the same as a normal period, where your body responds to production and release of an egg with certain hormone changes.

Birth control pills will regulate your menstrual cycles, but the effect normally lasts only as long as you take the pills. When you stop the pill, your periods may likely become irregular again.

The pills lowest in androgenic activity are most likely to help with additional symptoms such as hirsutism and acne as well as regulating your periods. Figuring out which oral contraceptive will work best based on the progestin it contains isn't always easy, though. Some birth control pills (such as desogestrel or levonorgestrel) have more androgenic activity than others.

But the amount of progestin in the pills also makes a difference; some pills may contain higher doses of progestins with less androgenic activity, decreasing the benefit. The best pill for symptoms of PCOS will have a progestin of low androgenic activity in a low dose. (See Table 7-2 for a list of different birth control pills, their composition, and their most common side effects.)

Many doctors prescribe Yasmin to women with PCOS because it contains an anti-testosterone agent, which can help alleviate some PCOS symptoms. Yasmin contains 3 milligrams of the progestin drospirenone, a derivative of aldactone (used as a diuretic), which has mild anti-androgenic activity.

Not all women can tolerate birth control pills; some women experience serious adverse reactions when they take them, especially weight gain and mood swings. Birth control pills also can increase your risk of developing blood clots and liver disorders; women over age 35 who smoke should not take birth control pills. Some women experience nausea while taking birth control pills; the vaginal ring or skin patch may prevent nausea.

Table 7-2	Common Birth Control Pills for PCOS		
Name	**Ingredients**	**Side Effects**	**Type of Pill**
Alesse-28	Ethinyl Estradiol 20 mcg; Levonorgestrel 0.10 mg	Headache, nausea, vomiting, breakthrough bleeding, acne	Higher androgenic, higher progestin, lower estrogen; monophasic
Demulen 1/35, Zovia 1/35 E	Ethinyl Estradiol 30 mcg; Ethynodiol diacetate 1 mg	Nausea, vomiting, weight gain	More progestogenic, low androgen; monophasic
Desogen	Ethinyl Estradiol 30 mcg; Desogetrel 0.15 mg	Headache, dizziness, nausea, breakthrough bleeding	Very low androgenic; monophasic
Levlen, Nodora, Nordette	Ethinyl Estradiol 30 mcg; Levonorgestrel 0.15 mg	Nausea, vomiting, spotting, weight gain, acne	Higher androgenic, higher progestin, lower estrogen; monophasic
Loestrin 1.5/30	Ethinyl Estradiol 30 mcg; Norethindrone acetate 1.5 mg	Acne, excess hair growth	Higher androgenic, higher progestin, lower estrogen; monophasic
Loestrin 1/20 Fe	Ethinyl Estradiol 20 mcg; Norethindrone acetate 1 mg	Acne, excess hair growth	More androgenic; monophasic

(continued)

Table 7-2 *(continued)*

Name	Ingredients	Side Effects	Type of Pill
Lo/Ovral	Ethinyl Estradiol 30 mcg; Norgestrel 0.3 mg	Nausea, vomiting	More progestogenic; monophasic
OrthoNovum 1/35	Ethinyl Estradiol 35 mcg; Noresthindrone acetate 1 mg	Headaches, nausea, mood changes	Higher estrogen, lower progestin; monophasic
Ortho Cyclen	Ethinyl estradiol 35 mcg; norgestimate 0.25 mg	Breast tenderness, mood changes, nausea	Lower progestin; monophasic
Yasmin	Ethinyl estradiol 30 mcg; Drospirenone 3.0 mg	May increase potassium levels; spotting, fluid retention, nausea	Anti-androgenic, higher progestogenic; monophasic

Treating Acne and Hairiness

Acne or excessive hairiness where you don't want it (called *hirsutism*) are usually due to your body producing too many male hormones (although all women make some). These symptoms can be distressing, because they're so visible when you look in the mirror. Fortunately, there are drugs that decrease these side effects.

Help from hormones

Oral contraceptive pills seem to work well for acne and hirsutism, as long as they contain an anti-androgen component. If you don't really want to or can't take a pill containing estrogen, ask your doctor for progestin-only pills.

If you take injectable progestins, your period can take up to a year to begin again, so you may want to consider oral methods instead if you're planning on trying to get pregnant in the near future. Like birth control pills, progestins alone can have side effects. Common ones include the following:

✔ **Weight gain:** Sometimes very difficult to lose (especially when taking the synthetic progestin medroxyprogesterone acetate [MPA], better known as Provera in its different forms). Because PCOS often causes weight gain all by itself, talk to your doctor about whether this is a good choice for you.

✔ **Depression and mood changes:** Can be potentially serious; if symptoms occur, ask your doctor about taking an antidepressant.

✔ **Irregular bleeding:** May subside after the first month or two.

✔ **Bone loss:** If you're on MPA, your doctor may test you periodically for a decrease in bone mineral density.

✔ **Decreased** *libido* (**sex drive**)

Table 7-3 lists common progestins and their dosages.

Table 7-3	Common Progestins and Their Dosages			
Drug	*Brand Name*	*Adminis- tration*	*Dose*	*Drawbacks*
Medroxy- progesterone acetate (MPA)	Depo-subQ Provera 104	Subcutan- eously	104 mg	Injection; can take up to a year to leave your system
MPA	Depo- Provera	Intra- muscular	100 mg to 150 mg every two to three months; can be more frequent in lesser dosages	Injection; can take up to a year to leave your system
MPA	Provera	Oral	10 mg to 60 mg daily	
Megestrol acetate	Megace	Oral	50 mg daily	
Norethindrone	Micronor	Oral	0.35 mg daily	
Norethindrone acetate	Aygestin, Norlutate	Oral	5 mg to 15 mg daily	

Other drugs that may help

Because metformin helps to reduce the levels of male hormones, it also may be useful in reducing hirsutism in PCOS.

New research has shown that statins may help to reduce androgen levels as well as correcting some of the metabolic symptoms associated with PCOS, such as elevated blood cholesterol levels.

Statins are medications that lower cholesterol levels either by decreasing the amount of cholesterol your body makes or by reducing the amount of cholesterol your body absorbs. However, more research is needed in this area before statins are generally prescribed for their testosterone-reducing properties.

Stopping Endometrial Buildup

By now you're undoubtedly beginning to realize that the same drugs can help treat a variety of conditions related to PCOS. The same birth control pills or progestins that keep your period regular and reduce symptoms of high male hormone levels also can keep your uterine lining from becoming too thick.

Building up the lining each month and then withdrawing progesterone so the lining is shed will decrease the risk of *endometrial hyperplasia,* a potentially dangerous condition that can increase your chances of developing uterine cancer. (See Chapter 9 for more about endometrial hyperplasia.)

Treating Weight Loss and Obesity

Weight gain — and difficulty losing it — is one of the most vexing issues of PCOS. Insulin resistance not only makes it hard to lose weight but can also increase your appetite. Talk about a catch-22. Prescription medications may help give you a jump-start with weight loss that will give you the impetus and encouragement to keep going on your own. Over-the-counter medications are a bit trickier — *buyer beware* is always a safe bet when trying supplements (with a few exceptions).

Prescription drug treatment

Losing weight can help PCOS in a number of ways, not the least of which is a boost in your self-esteem. Drugs seem like a nice easy answer to how to lose weight painlessly, but be aware that weight-loss drugs, in most cases, are no miracle cure.

The idea of drugs for weight loss is that they can give you a boost in helping you overcome a weight-loss plateau. They can't be taken indefinitely, so sooner or later you always have to go back to dieting and exercising.

Nevertheless, a number of prescription drugs can give you a weight-loss boost to get you started.

Opting for orlistat

This drug, sold as Xenical in the United States, stops you from absorbing about one-third of the fat that you eat. Because fat is so energy-dense (9 calories per gram), you can stop a lot of calories from being absorbed using this drug. However, don't expect to be able to continue eating lots of fatty food — oh, no!

Unless you also cut down on the amount of fat you eat, the unabsorbed fat simply leaks out of you in a rather embarrassing and smelly way! The gut can cope with passing a little undigested fat, but not too much. You may lose some of your fat-soluble vitamins such as vitamin A, D, and E with this drug, too, so your diet must supply adequate amounts of these vitamins.

An over-the-counter form of this drug that contains half the dose of the prescription form, called Alli, cuts fat absorption by around 25 percent but has the same side effects if you eat too much fat. According to the manufacturer, you can safely eat around 15 grams of fat per meal before symptoms appear.

Even a low dose of this drug can be effective if combined with a weight-loss diet. In addition to significant weight loss, you may experience a resultant drop in blood pressure and a decrease in the harmful blood fat levels. Normally, you can't stay on orlistat for longer than two years.

Phentermine for weight loss

Phentermine, sold commercially as prescription Adipex-P oral and Ionamin, was once half of a very popular off-label diet drug combination commonly called Fen-Phen (fenfluramine and phentermine combined). Phentermine is a sympathomimetic amine; it works by suppressing appetite, although it's not clear why it works.

Fen-Phen was taken off the market when a number of people developed heart-valve disease and pulmonary hypertension. Fenfluramine was taken off the market, too, but phentermine is still available as a prescription drug. Phentermine is usually prescribed for a period of three to six weeks.

Common side effects of phentermine include the following:

- ✔ Constipation
- ✔ Diarrhea
- ✔ Dry mouth
- ✔ Unpleasant taste in the mouth
- ✔ Vomiting

More serious side effects include the following:

- ✔ Anxiety
- ✔ Chest pain
- ✔ Dizziness
- ✔ Feeling like your heart is pounding
- ✔ Fluid retention and swelling
- ✔ High blood pressure
- ✔ Increased heart rate
- ✔ Muscle weakness
- ✔ Restlessness

Notify your doctor immediately if any of these side effects occur.

In addition, some people have developed an addiction to or dependency on this medication. Withdrawal symptoms such as depression or fatigue can develop if you suddenly stop taking the medication.

Going over the counter

The dietary supplements business is a multi-billion-dollar business; according to the Office of Dietary Supplements (part of the National Institutes of Health), Americans spent over $20 billion on supplements of various kinds in 2004. Over 50 percent of Americans use some type of dietary supplement each year. There's no limit to the types of over-the-counter weight-loss products available, from homeopathic extracts, to pills, to potions in the form of meal replacement shakes and diet bars.

Meal replacement drinks and diet bars, where you substitute a diet supplement for a meal, tend to be the least harmful. Most herbs and other supplements, despite their lavish promises, don't deliver any real weight loss.

Although many of the more dangerous herbs and supplements have now been banned, you may still find them turning up for sale in some places, including on the Internet. Many more potentially dangerous compounds still lurk out there, and even supplements that aren't dangerous to your health can be harmful to your pocketbook.

The banned ones were based on dangerous drugs such as amphetamines and ephedra (also known as ma huang); both drugs can lead to heart problems and death. Recently some of the weight-loss herbals have been found to lead to liver toxicity.

A recent article in a scientific journal claimed that the use of performance-enhancing and weight-loss supplements is prevalent in the United States. These drugs are the kind taken by athletes to keep their weight down and their athletic abilities high. However, they also can be taken by someone desperate to lose weight. The article reports a great deal of concern about the side effects of such supplements, including the information that the particularly risky ones to look out for are the caffeine-based herbal supplements because they can cause blood pressure to rise to dangerously high levels.

Many of the supplements sold today are particularly tricky to assess because they consist of not one ingredient, but many mixed together. If you have a bad reaction, you won't know which herb or supplement caused it. Many have names that sound very similar to prescription drugs.

Because over-the-counter supplements change frequently, a detailed list is hard to keep current. Here are some of the favored supplements at the time of this writing:

- ✔ **Acai:** The acai berry, which comes from the Brazilian Amazon region, is a berry high in antioxidants. Proponents claim that acai is a "superfood" with weight-loss properties as well as a number of other health benefits.

- ✔ **Chromium:** Chromium sold as chromium picolinate is a perennial diet favorite. This mineral may enhance insulin sensitivity, which can lead to weight loss.

- ✔ **Green tea:** Fans of green tea claim it increases *thermogenesis,* or heat production. Green tea contains caffeine, which can speed your metabolism in large amounts, although with unpleasant side effects.

- ✔ **Hoodia:** A cactus-like plant, this African drug claims to have potent appetite-suppressant properties that work by tricking the brain into thinking you're full. Because the effective and safe limits of hoodia haven't been established, it's difficult to know if the product you buy will have any effect — or too much.

- ✔ **Yohimbe:** Made from the bark of the evergreen tree, yohimbe or the chemical it contains, called *yohimbine,* is a central nervous system stimulant that increases fat mobilization and decreases fat stores. Like most supplements, no safe and effective dose has been established.

These over-the-counter supplements are not rigorously tested by medical experts in a controlled study and not approved by the FDA. Claims are often based on hearsay, small numbers of uncontrolled people with no common basis, or even exaggeration. Their claims are almost always found to be unsubstantiated in real clinical trials, most often being the same as a placebo and sometimes having a negative effect.

Chapter 8

Giving Alternative Treatments a Shot

. . . .

In This Chapter

▶ Supplementing your way through PCOS

▶ Adding herbs to treat PCOS

▶ Seeing if complementary therapies work for you

▶ Being cautious about alternative diets

. . . .

Diagnosing and treating PCOS has come a long way in the last few years, but there's still no cure for PCOS. Doctors know how to treat PCOS to keep symptoms at bay. And much of the treatment lies in your hands. By adopting a holistic approach (following the right diet and lifestyle), PCOS can become virtually symptomless.

However, the growth in understanding of PCOS is not helped by people who claim wondrous cures that, at best, can disappoint you and at worst do some real harm.

This chapter looks at alternative treatments that have been advocated for PCOS, giving you the lowdown on whether these treatments are helpful, dangerous, or likely to do nothing.

Supplements: Taking Care not to Overdo It

The best way for you to achieve peak vitamin and mineral status is by eating a wide variety of foods. However, if your diet has been poor or restricted to less than 1,500 calories for some reason, you may need a full-spectrum multivitamin and mineral supplement. In the case of calcium and iron, a little extra in the diet in the form of a supplement may be beneficial in PCOS.

Supplements are not a cure, but they can be a valuable part of your overall strategy to fight PCOS. However, supplements are not harmless, and in some cases they can be seriously harmful. With supplements, the old adage that if a little is good, a lot is better does not apply.

You can overdose on supplements, especially if you're taking supplements from several different sources or taking blends of different herbs. Treat supplements exactly as you do drugs, because they can have powerful effects on the body. With some supplements, the difference between a level that's just right (the recommended daily amount, or RDA) and a toxic level can be quite small.

Dietary supplements aren't as well regulated as prescription medications in the United States. The purity and exact dosage may vary from brand to brand and even bottle to bottle in the same brand. Only buy from well-known companies that have the United States Pharmacopeia (USP) seal.

Vitamin A

Vitamin A, a fat-soluble vitamin, is necessary for the maintenance of healthy skin and hormonal balance, which has led some people to claim that taking vitamin A in the diet, or as a supplement, helps with some PCOS symptoms.

The evidence is still lacking, but you do need to make sure that you're getting an adequate amount of vitamin A in your diet, and this aim is best achieved by ensuring that you take a good range of the following foods:

- ✔ Liver (but avoid it if you're planning to get pregnant or are already pregnant)
- ✔ Carrots
- ✔ Leafy green vegetables
- ✔ Yellow and orange fruits

Carrots, leafy green vegetables, and yellow and orange fruits are sources of carotenoids such as beta-carotene, some of which are converted into vitamin A in the body. They're a safe source of vitamin A because you can't as easily overdose on carotenoids as you can on animal sources such as liver, which contain very large amounts of vitamin A — and if you do, the consequences aren't so serious. (You may, however, turn orange!)

If you decide to take a supplement containing vitamin A, never exceed the RDA because high-dose supplements taken long term can lead to osteoporosis. Furthermore, high doses taken at around the time of conception have been shown to increase the risk of birth defects in the baby. So, make sure that you have enough vitamin A in your diet, but not too much. Because vitamin A is fat-soluble, it's stored in the body, which makes overdose symptoms more likely if you take too much.

Vitamin B6

Traditionally, B6 is the vitamin used to treat PMS symptoms such as acne. However, the doses recommended in some studies were at levels up to 100 times the RDA. Experts now say that a maximum of 10 mg a day of vitamin B6 should be consumed, but such a dose is unlikely to have any effect on the symptoms of PCOS.

 Only take doses greater than 10 mg per day under medical supervision, because vitamin B6 can cause nerve damage when taken in high doses.

B6 is found in a variety of meats, poultry, fish, fortified cereals, beans, and some fruits and vegetables.

Calcium and vitamin D

Some evidence suggests that altered hormone levels in PCOS can lead to a loss of calcium from the bones; calcium loss can lead to low bone density and osteoporosis. This loss is similar to that in women who have gone through menopause (either naturally or due to having their ovaries removed).

Recent evidence also has shown that women with a high intake of vitamin D and calcium appear to have a lower risk of developing type 2 diabetes. Both nutrients seem to play a role in improving insulin production and sensitivity.

To get the calcium you need, consume three to four servings of milk-based foods every day. One serving is

- ✔ Five ounces of yogurt
- ✔ Around 6 ounces of milk
- ✔ One ounce of cheese

Manufacturers have stepped up to the plate in creating low-fat versions of dairy products traditionally high in fat. You can find low-fat versions of yogurt, cream cheese, cheese, and milk, not to mention milkshakes made with low-fat milk.

If you want to use some full-fat cheese for extra flavor in a dish, you'll pile on fewer calories if you use a strong-flavored cheese and grate it to make it go further.

Don't avoid dairy products with the mistaken belief that they're high in calories. However, if you need to avoid milk and milk products for allergy reasons, you can use soy alternatives — just be sure to buy the calcium-fortified versions.

If you have lactose intolerance, as many American adults do, you can buy dairy products containing *lactase,* the enzyme that breaks down *lactose,* the sugar that causes gastrointestinal symptoms in people who lack lactase. If you'd rather drink regular milk, buy lactase drops to add to milk or take oral lactase supplements with meals to prevent symptoms.

If you really don't like using lactase drops, then you'll need to take a daily calcium supplement that provides you with 100 percent of your RDA.

Vitamin D sources are more limited but can be found in

- ✔ Oily fish (or fish oil supplements)
- ✔ Eggs
- ✔ Fortified spreads
- ✔ Fortified breakfast cereals

Iron

Although absent or infrequent periods are common in PCOS, you may be one of the less common PCOS sufferers who experience very heavy, prolonged, or more-frequent-than-monthly periods. If this is the case, you may find that such loss of blood causes a drain on your iron reserves.

You need to take care to get enough iron in your diet; otherwise, you may develop iron-deficiency anemia. Symptoms of anemia include fatigue, pallor, and shortness of breath during physical activity.

Iron supplements can cause constipation and stomach upset. So getting your iron from food is best unless your doctor tells you to take a prescribed supplement. Good sources of iron include

- Beef
- Pork
- Sardines
- Fortified breakfast cereals
- Beans
- Lentils
- Green vegetables
- Dried fruit

Iron from animal sources, called *heme iron,* is better absorbed than iron from plant sources.

 To absorb the maximum amount of iron from non-meat sources, eat it with a source of vitamin C (such as fruit juice, a green vegetable, or citrus fruit), or take heme and non-heme iron sources together in the same meal.

Zinc

Zinc is thought to help hormone-related acne and is believed to work best when coupled with adequate vitamin A in the diet. Some researchers believe that a lack of zinc in the diet leads to an increased production of *androgens* (male hormones), and because PCOS is already associated with an increase in androgens, you don't need any more!

Zinc is best obtained from dietary sources because zinc supplements may interfere with the absorption of other minerals from the gut. Dietary sources of zinc include

- Beef
- Pork
- Lamb
- Peanuts
- Brazil nuts
- Whole-grain cereals
- Pumpkin seeds
- Yeast

Chromium

Overt chromium deficiency produces symptoms of diabetes and insulin resistance. Modern diets, with their reliance on refined grains, especially if also high in sugar, may result in marginal chromium deficiency. You may read claims that chromium supplements help with weight loss and muscle buildup, but such claims have never been proven in mainstream research. Chromium helps insulin to work efficiently and an adequate amount in the diet may help in reducing insulin resistance.

Chromium supplements on their own (rather than in a multivitamin) aren't recommended because a fine line exists between taking a safe amount of chromium and overdosing. Some cases have been reported where people taking regular doses of a supplement that provided more than the recommended intake developed liver and kidney failure.

To be safe, all you need to do is follow the balanced low-GI diet advocated in Chapter 4. This diet provides you naturally with plenty of the foods that are high in chromium, such as

- Beef
- Liver
- Eggs
- Chicken
- Whole grains
- Bran cereals
- Wheat germ (available in jars and in whole-grain bread)
- Green peppers
- Tomatoes
- Onions
- Apples
- Bananas
- Spinach

Essential fatty acids

Essential fatty acids are deemed "essential" because your body needs them but can't make them on its own. If you eat a balanced diet that includes a wide variety of food, you normally get these essential fatty acids from oils that you consume.

You actually require two types of fatty acids: One is an omega-3 called alpha-linolenic acid, and the other is an omega-6 called linoleic acid. After these get into the bloodstream, they're converted into a myriad of important chemicals in the body.

When incorporated into the diet, oils containing a high level of essential fatty acids are believed to help reduce insulin resistance and improve glucose metabolism. Some people claim they can even help acne because they have a balancing action on hormones.

Fish oils can help lower cholesterol and triglyceride levels, which can reduce the risk of developing heart disease. They also may decrease blood clotting that can lead to stroke.

Sources of essential fatty acids include vegetables, nuts, seeds, oils, and oily fish. You need to have a varied source of these every day in your diet. Getting adequate omega-3 fatty acids can be hard if you don't eat oily fish, in which case you may need a fish oil supplement.

Taking a Leaf from Herbal Medicine

A lot has been claimed for herbal medicines in the treatment of PCOS. The truth is that the evidence is still very sparse. If herbs really got half the results some advocates attribute to them, they would be recommended by doctors everywhere, and news about them would travel like wildfire among PCOS sufferers.

If you do want to try herbs, stick to the ones listed here. Other herbal supplements actually may do more harm than good, and cases of liver damage are not unheard of with some questionable herbal preparations.

See a qualified medical herbalist if you want to try a variety of herbal remedies. If you're on any other medication or you're trying for a baby or are pregnant or breastfeeding, double-check with your doctor to make sure that taking the herbal supplement is safe.

Agnus Castus

Agnus Castus is also known as chasteberry (because it was used by monks to reduce any horny feelings they may have had, or so the rumors go!), monk's pepper, or Abraham's balm. Agnus Castus is the dried berry extract from a densely branched shrub that grows in the Mediterranean and central Asia. You can easily buy the supplement in pharmacies or health-food stores these days, and it's available as a powdered form made into tablets or capsules or as a concentrated liquid herbal extract. This herbal extract claims to help relieve many PCOS symptoms, including anovulation.

When you take Agnus Castus, a whole cascade is set into motion: First, the extract exerts a hormonal effect via the pituitary gland in the brain. Then the pituitary gland releases a hormone that stimulates the ovaries to produce more luteinizing hormone (LH) and less follicle-stimulating hormone (FSH). The result is that the balance of estrogen to progesterone is changed in favor of progesterone.

Agnus Castus is also effective in reducing PMS symptoms. In Germany, where many herbs are government regulated and approved, this herb is approved for the regulation of hormone levels, so something may really be in this herb that works.

The recommended dose is 40 mg of dried extract, 40 drops of liquid extract, or 175 mg to 200 mg in capsule form daily.

And don't worry, no evidence exists that it helps promote chastity in women!

Saw Palmetto

Saw Palmetto may help reduce hirsutism, but the evidence is still weak. Saw Palmetto supposedly reduces the level of circulating testosterone (an androgen), which reduces hirsutism.

Traditionally this herb is used as a boost to the male reproductive system and as a treatment for prostate problems, but don't let that put you off! No side effects have been documented with this herbal preparation, but there's also no long-term research on it.

Other herbals

Other herbals sometimes recommended for use in PCOS include the following:

- **False unicorn root:** A Native American remedy for menstrual irregularities.
- **Licorice:** Used to reduce androgen levels and improve the LH:FSH ratio, as well as to regulate hormones; often combined with white peony, which also is said to reduce elevated testosterone levels.

✔ **Dong quai:** Used to regulate the menstrual cycle; dubbed the "ultimate herb" for women. Dong quai has blood-thinning properties; don't take it if you have very heavy periods.

✔ **Blue cohosh:** Used as a uterine and ovarian tonic. It can cause fetal heart defects, so don't take it if you're pregnant.

✔ **Motherwort:** Used to regulate the menstrual cycle and improve blood flow.

✔ **Nettle:** Considered to be a uterine tonic.

Some of these herbals claim to have a progestogenic action in the body to counter high androgen levels, whereas others are meant to improve the skin or help the liver efficiently metabolize hormones. However, evidence for these herbs actually achieving these functions tends to be anecdotal.

Trying Complementary Therapies

Complementary therapies complement or offer an alternative to traditional medical practice and treatment and are unregulated by medical authorities. If nothing else, complementary therapies can be relaxing and act as a real feel-good factor in your armor against PCOS.

Unfortunately, evidence on the success of complementary therapies in PCOS tends to be anecdotal rather than science-based. Of course, the defenders of complementary therapies may tell you that's because research money is available only for testing drugs (because testing is paid for by the big pharmaceutical companies who have little interest in testing "natural" therapies, which hold little profit margin for them). So, the debate rages on. . . .

Complementary therapies should be used as an adjunct to mainstream treatment. Don't shun the medical profession and just seek help from the complementary side, because you may not get adequate treatment for certain symptoms that, if left unchecked, can lead to long-term problems, including uncontrolled blood sugar (which can result in blindness and kidney damage if not treated) and absent periods (which can give rise to endometrial cancer).

Some complementary therapies, and what they claim to deliver, are shown in Table 8-1.

Table 8-1 Complementary Therapies Claimed to be Helpful in PCOS

Therapy	What It Claims to Offer	What to Watch Out For
Acupuncture (the insertion of small needles at various key points on the body)	Kick-starts periods.	Requires that you're treated for one week or more every month.
Aromatherapy (involves massaging essential oils into the body and sometimes additionally burning them in a vaporizer)	Balances the hormones.	Long-term treatment is usually advocated.
Herbalism (using certain medical herbs to treat symptoms)	Encourages hormonal balance and is a treatment for many PCOS symptoms. May be advised as an adjunct to diet and lifestyle changes.	Seek out a properly qualified herbalist or you may receive herbs that are harmful. Don't use as an alternative to proper medical treatment.
Nutrition therapy (advocating dietary changes and use of supplements)	Claims to match a diet to your unique problems and circumstances.	Nutritional therapists are not dietitians and have rarely received the same standards of training. They usually advocate supplements, often in doses that are far too high.
Homeopathy (the use of almost undetectable amounts of chemicals, which are meant to stimulate the body to heal itself)	A homeopath takes a detailed history and chooses a unique treatment for each individual. Individual PCOS symptoms can be targeted.	Long-term treatment is advocated because it may take up to six months to see a lessening of symptoms.
Reflexology (the stimulation of specific reflex points in the foot that are thought to link to energy channels throughout the body)	Claimed to help regulate the menstrual cycle and aid relaxation.	No downside except for cost and the fact that it may set up false hopes.

Avoiding Alternative Diets

Alternative diets are "niche" diets that claim to eradicate your PCOS symptoms. They may not follow the usual rules on healthy eating, which is to eat a variety of foods, to have low-GI carbs, and to limit fat and salt. This section helps you to analyze these diets for what they are.

Low-carb diets

A low-carbohydrate diet contains a much smaller percentage of carbohydrate calories than the 50 percent recommended by bona-fide experts (see Chapter 3). On these diets you have to cut down or cut out foods such as potatoes, pasta, rice, and bread, along with foods containing sugar, and possibly fruit too.

As far as weight loss is concerned, some short-term success may be gained in following a low-carb diet, but no real data show the long-term success of such diets. Here's why these diets may work in the short term:

✔ By following such a diet, you're cutting out a large food group and, thus, restricting the number of foods you're allowed to eat, which means you eat fewer calories. Naturally, you get bored eating fewer kinds of food, eat less of them, and lose weight!

✔ By cutting down carbs, you tend to eat more protein (along with more fat). Some evidence exists that a higher protein intake helps to curb your appetite.

✔ On such a diet, you tend to produce high levels of ketones as a result of the body trying to metabolize fat, especially in the first two weeks of the diet. High ketone levels can lead to feelings of nausea and subsequent loss of appetite.

But the real reason you shouldn't follow a low-carb diet is that the disadvantages (from a health point of view) outweigh the advantages. Here are just two of the disadvantages:

✔ You eat a lot of fat on such a diet, which may increase your risk of getting heart disease.

✔ Ketones are highly toxic to newly conceived babies, so if you become pregnant on such a diet, you're putting your baby at risk.

Get medical advice before committing yourself to any low-carb diet, including the Atkins diet, the Carbohydrate Addict's diet, Protein Power, Sugar Busters, or the Zone. Some of them are more severe (and, therefore, potentially more dangerous) than others.

Detox diets

Detox diets claim to be the answer to everything these days and carry with them some magical air — probably because no one really knows what the diets are all about or how they work, other than they somehow rid the body of stuff that shouldn't be there.

Detox diets tend to involve eating only a very narrow range of foods. Limiting the range of foods consumed can lead to some weight loss, but you shouldn't stay on this sort of diet for more than a few days; the gains to your health and weight loss tend to be small. PCOS sufferers with big appetites, who regularly feel the effects of low blood sugar, are likely to feel, frankly, awful on such a restricted diet.

The body has organs that deal with waste and toxins. The kidney filters and cleans the blood perfectly well in most people, and the liver does a great detoxifying job, as long as you don't overload it too often (such as with regular bouts of binge drinking).

However, the body prefers not to have to cope with unnecessary problems so don't imbibe too much alcohol and stay off any unnecessary drugs. If you do overtax your liver, a detox diet is unlikely to be the solution to reverse the damage.

Avoid products that claim to detox, especially if they claim to enhance the immune system, relieve pain, flush out toxins, and stimulate circulation. These products are very unlikely to have undergone proper medical tests, and such claims are allowed only after rigorous medical testing.

Organic or additive/caffeine/ alcohol-free diets

Some diets work by making you feel guilty for eating ordinary food bought from the supermarket that may not have been organically grown, and that may include the odd cup of tea or coffee and the occasional glass of wine. Just to reassure you, nothing's wrong with doing so!

Many of the books and articles on PCOS contain "information" to make you feel very guilty. For example, some diets insist that you have to go organic and avoid every last food dye or additive. Even that nice cup of tea or the odd glass of wine are guaranteed to evoke guilt. Most of these diets don't cause any physical harm (just mental anguish!), but they're unlikely to do you any good either. They're more likely to increase your stress and leave you unable to cope. Thinking about trying to eat a balanced diet and avoid weight gain is hard enough, let alone having to make sure that everything you consume is additive-free and organic.

For a start, organic food is expensive and not always readily available. Most nutrition experts claim that eating organic doesn't make you any healthier, but feel free to buy it if you think it tastes better or if you want to support sustainable farming. Similarly, the additives in food are often there for good reasons, such as keeping food fresh and reducing bacterial growth. Before being used in food, additives have to undergo rigorous testing, so they come with a clean bill of health with regards to human safety.

Of course, your diet is probably more nutritious if you buy as many fresh ingredients as possible and don't rely too much on ready-made meals, which often contain excessive salt, sugar, and trans fats.

Chapter 9

Balancing Body, Mind, and Spirit

*T*o achieve maximum results when trying to improve your health, you need to balance the whole body, both mentally and physically. Looking at diet and exercise while ignoring the state of your mind won't give the results you want.

This chapter looks at how to psych yourself up for the challenge of reducing your PCOS symptoms. We help you motivate yourself to stick to a diet and exercise regime while staying stress free.

Psyching Up for the Task

Like any task, changing your diet and lifestyle isn't something that you can launch straight into. You have several stages to go through before you get on with it. In this section, we list the eight steps of a reasonable plan to help you change your lifestyle. We also give you tips for staying positive and setting realistic goals.

Following the eight-point plan

Here's a quick eight-point plan for changing your diet and/ or lifestyle:

1. **Decide why you feel that you need to change your diet, lifestyle, or both.**

2. **Decide what changes you need to make.**

3. **Make a list of the advantages and disadvantages of changing.**

   Do the advantages outweigh the disadvantages? If the answer is yes, then get going on your goals! If you hit a low point later on, you can refer back to the list and see just why you need to stick to your plan!

   If no, you may need to go back and rethink the list in a few weeks, because you're likely to fail if you try to force changes on your life without being wholeheartedly behind them.

4. **Figure out when to start.**

   Your doctor may have told you that you need to do something immediately for the sake of your health. But you may want to put it off until you've had time to think things through, or until a big event (like a vacation or a wedding) is over. Don't put it off longer than a week or so if you've been told to do something urgently or if you really feel that something needs to be done.

5. **Assemble all the tools you need for the job ahead.**

   The tools can include having the knowledge about what to do, getting rid of foods in your house that aren't conducive to the new diet, and buying suitable alternatives.

6. **Improve the skills you need for the job ahead.**

   If you're useless in the kitchen, learn how to cook (it can be fun — honest!) by reading cookbooks, watching television cooking programs, or signing up for a cooking course. If you don't have a clue where to start to plan an exercise program, read Chapter 6. You may even want to sign up with a personal trainer — just one session with a trainer can point you in the right direction.

7. **Make plans and contingency plans.**

   If you're changing your routine to include exercise, figure out where it'll fit into your day. You also need to have some sort of a diet plan to follow. Plan out your food intake and recipes at least two to three days in advance, and then check that you have the necessary food ingredients for each meal. Think ahead to plan how to handle going out for dinner, celebrating holidays, or other special occasions.

8. **Think about providing yourself with motivational support.**

   You may have to tell friends and family how you'd like them to support you (such as asking them not to buy you chocolates). Most people want to help, but they can't read your mind, so tell them. Plan certain rewards for each milestone (such as a massage, new jewelry, or clothes). Dieting with a friend helps you motivate each other. If you really struggle with motivation on your own, consider a regular personal trainer or some sort of motivational counseling sessions. You may benefit from a weight-loss group, such as Weight Watchers, or from a few visits with a private dietitian.

Before starting any sort of diet or exercise regime, talk to your doctor. He may be able to refer you to a suitable therapist (such as a dietitian, occupational therapist, or physiotherapist) who can give you some tailored advice about what's best for you.

Staying positive

Believing that you're going to succeed is half the battle. The eight-point plan in the preceding section gives you a framework to get ready and motivated for change, but these additional motivators also may help.

Break a big task down into small, manageable chunks

Whatever your goal is — to lose 30 pounds or to get to the gym three times a week — it can seem like a mammoth task. Keep two things in mind when the huge mountain looming in front of you seems insurmountable:

- **Take the first step.** A Chinese proverb says that a journey of a thousand miles begins with a single step. After you've made that first step, the next one is easier to make, and then the next one, and before you know it, you're well on your way.

- **Break up the task into bite-size steps, and then reward yourself for achieving each step.** Set some realistic timelines of when you expect to achieve each small goal. With a weight loss of 30 pounds, aim for 5 pounds at a time. Your reward needs to be something that helps you to feel good about yourself (such as a haircut or facial) or that you enjoy (such as a trip to the movies or a new piece of jewelry). Avoid rewarding yourself with food!

Don't let failure keep you down

Because you're human, you make mistakes and fail from time to time. The secret of coping with failure is to understand that it does happen and not to let it drag you down for long. Shake yourself off mentally, and start again. Table 9-1 lists some common causes of failure and advice for overcoming them so that you don't lose motivation.

Table 9-1 Ways to Stick to Your Weight-Loss Goals

Problem	Solution
Setting daunting goals that seem impossible to achieve, such as a total of 100 pounds to lose.	Break up the task into smaller chunks, each with an achievable milestone that doesn't take longer than a month.
Feeling disappointed and losing motivation when you've followed your diet carefully and done your physical activity, yet no weight loss results.	Weight does plateau from time to time, and you should see it falling again soon. If it doesn't, then you may need to write down everything you eat, being honest with portion sizes and every last nibble. Take a good, hard look to see if you really are sticking to the diet you set out to follow. From time to time, it's also a good idea to change up your exercise routine to give your body a jump-start.
Drifting back into your old comforting ways of eating what you like and doing no exercise.	Look at the reasons you wrote down for why you wanted to improve your diet and lifestyle. Don't let a few lapsed days sidetrack you. Just shake yourself off and get back on track!
Repeatedly slipping up and failing.	Check that you haven't been too rigid with your goals and that you haven't set yourself up for failure.

Keep a journal

The act of writing down the things that you want to achieve, and how you can achieve them, is psychologically positive. Committing your objectives and long- and short-term plans to paper helps you feel like you're well on your journey.

Keep a log of your progress, such as what exercises you've done, your weight, your waist measurement, and so on; this log enables you to see your progress. If you're going through a negative patch, you can see how well you've done in the past and how you encountered hard times before and came through them.

Chapter 4 explains how to keep a food diary, in which you list absolutely everything that you eat and drink, when and where you ate them, and how you felt when eating them. This kind of record-keeping enables you to build up a picture of why you eat and whether a pattern emerges that may need to be broken. For example, a bad day at work may result in your raiding the cookie jar when you get home. When you know your triggers, you can plan ahead to thwart them.

Clear out the negative energy

You don't need negativity in your life because it tends to drag you down with it. Clear out negativity in the following ways:

✔ **Avoid friends who get jealous because they may not want you to succeed and may try to bring you down if they see you doing well.** Some friends and loved ones may be worried that you're going to change from the person they know if you're successful. Talk to them honestly about what it means to you to make these changes.

✔ **You don't need to get all fanatical about feng shui, but the idea behind this philosophy makes a lot of sense.** Create a sense of space around you and have your surroundings obey some kind of order. You may find that when you de-clutter your surroundings you have more energy, are less stressed, and are able to concentrate more on the job at hand. See for yourself how freeing and motivating a weekend clearing out the junk can be; you may find that you then want to clear out the junk from your own diet and lifestyle. And don't make it just a one-off exercise — take steps to ensure that it doesn't build up to the same level of clutter again!

   If you want to find out more about feng shui, check out *Feng Shui For Dummies,* by David Daniel Kennedy (Wiley).

✔ **Make sure that your doctor or any therapist you use isn't filling you with frightening thoughts, or trying to lecture you about what you should be doing.** You need someone who can fill you with hope and inspiration. Try having a word with her or simply ask to see someone else.

✔ **Lack of money can be a very negative influence, so try to sort out some sort of budget so that your income doesn't exceed your outgo.** If necessary, see a financial adviser.

✔ **Lack of time is another negative influence; continually chasing your tail is very stressful.** Making time for yourself is a bit like physically de-cluttering your life; you need to think about what you do each day and each week and whether anything can be dropped. You may need to become more self-centered and say no to certain things.

✔ **If other worries are playing on your mind, you aren't going to be in a positive mood for moving ahead on your diet and lifestyle plan.** Writing down your worries or sharing them with someone else can help. Part of the new you is to tackle your worries and concerns head on and see if they can be overcome. Don't do this all at once, but prioritize your "worry" list and deal with the top priorities first.

Talk nicely to yourself

According to recent research, approximately 87 percent of people talk to themselves as if they were their most despicable enemy. If they don't know something, they call themselves "stupid"; if they drop something, they call themselves "clumsy"; and so on. This sort of negative-speak develops into a self-fulfilling prophecy.

Start to talk positively about yourself and give yourself permission to succeed and you probably will. For example, "I have strong willpower, so I can resist that gooey cake with my coffee" is much more motivating than "I'm a fatty — I'll never lose weight." Even if no one else has faith in you, you must have faith in yourself. Who knows? You may even find that other people catch on to your positive attitude about yourself.

When the challenge seems too great, have some positive-affirmation statements that you can repeat to yourself posted in large writing around your house and work. Here are some examples:

- ✔ "I'm looking and feeling good."
- ✔ "My diet is healthy and doing me good."
- ✔ "I like exercising because it makes me feel good."
- ✔ "Every day I'm one step closer to my goal."

You can create your own affirmations, but they have to be positive and in the present tense.

Being realistic

No one said that changing your diet and lifestyle is going to be easy. No change is easy. When you do something in a particular way for a period of time, your neural pathways get set into doing things a set way, and the longer you spend doing them a certain way, the more entrenched those patterns become and the harder it is to change them. So, if you always have a cookie when you have a cup of tea or coffee, you almost get to depend on having that cookie and you really notice the loss when you don't have it.

To break out of this cycle, you have to reprogram the pathway. The longer you do something in a different way, the more the old links get broken and you find doing things the new way habitual. This can work for everything from not piling your plate with food to not having dessert to always walking up the stairs rather than taking the elevator.

Of course, things aren't that simple, because other factors come into play. If you start cutting down on food and get ravenously hungry midmorning, no amount of neural reprogramming is going to convince you not to have that doughnut with your cup of coffee, unless you have a backup choice handy.

The Holistic Balancing Act

The term *holistic* means being concerned about the whole person, instead of focusing on different parts of the body or mind. PCOS affects your whole body, including your state of mind. In PCOS, the symptoms are all related and often have a common cause that you can tackle when you see the bigger picture.

You can't isolate what's going on in one part of your life from the rest of your life. Although putting certain aspects of your life on hold for a while is fine (for example, forgetting about that argument with your partner when you need to focus at work), sooner or later you have to deal with this part of your life. So, if something isn't quite right in one part of your life, whether it be physical or emotional, it can affect the rest of you and your body. Equally, if something is going really well in one bit, it can give your whole body a lift. Have you noticed that you can be feeling really awful one day, and then you get some really good news and suddenly life is rosy again and you feel physically so much better?

This section shows you how you can balance the physical along with the mental parts of your life.

Physical well-being

You may feel that the physical manifestations of PCOS symptoms are turning you into a wreck, but you can do a lot to improve your physical well-being right now, including your external appearance:

✔ **Take a long, hard look at what's in your wardrobe.** The general rule is to prune out anything that you haven't worn for a year. If something is too small for you, it does no good to say that you're going to keep it until it fits, because all it does is serve as a constant reminder of how you've failed. All your clothes in your wardrobe should flatter you physically. If they don't, go shopping. You don't need loads of clothes, just some good-quality separates that you can mix and match and that work for you. If you're not sure what suits you, see an image consultant. Go with a friend to make it more fun!

✔ **Stand tall and be aware of your posture.** Good posture is flattering to your figure and prevents you from getting aches and pains. Like any new habit, the more you practice good posture, the more it becomes second nature.

✔ **Do some physical activity whenever you get the chance.** Even short bouts of ten minutes that get your heart rate up are beneficial. You immediately feel better, physically and mentally.

✔ **Change your image.** You don't have to go in for the full makeover thing (although having advice from an image consultant is a great treat), but you may want to try a new haircut, or try wearing an outfit you wouldn't normally wear. You can even invest in some snazzy sunglasses.

✔ **Get treatment for your PCOS.** Don't put it off. If you feel the treatment isn't working, ask the experts why and find out what you need to be doing instead.

People with medical conditions often feel they're powerless and that their lives have been taken over by visits to doctors, being monitored, taking medications, and so on. However, with PCOS, you can do a lot to help yourself. So, don't be a spectator of your own treatment; take back the reins and feel empowered and motivated by what you can actually do for yourself. *Remember:* All you're doing is to try to eat healthily and get some exercise, something everyone should be doing!

Perceiving that your physical appearance doesn't live up to what you think society expects women to look like can be a real cause of low self-esteem, particularly in teenagers and younger women. If you feel under this pressure, don't resort to extreme tactics such as starving yourself. Extreme behavior tends to give rise to more extreme problems. Bulimia nervosa is more common in women with PCOS than in women without it. (For information on eating disorders and PCOS, refer to Chapter 4.)

Mental well-being

Self-esteem is a vicious cycle: The less you have of it, the less likely you are to pull yourself up by your bootstraps and work on yourself so that you can improve your self-esteem. On the other hand, if you do start making changes, you get positive feedback; making gradual improvements to your diet and health makes you feel better about yourself, and that makes you want to continue to make those changes that make you feel good!

Here are some tips on how to psych yourself up mentally into believing in yourself and feeling good about yourself:

✔ **Think about what you're good at — and not only work-related stuff.** Write them down. Perhaps you're good at painting, being a good listener, or remembering people's birthdays. The next time you need a reminder about who you are and what you can achieve, take a look at this list.

✔ **Ask people you know and trust to make lists of what they think you excel at and why they like you.** This can give you some pleasant surprises. Don't ask them to write out lists of your less-pleasant attributes — at least not until you have an ego the size of a planet!

✔ **Find out how to be assertive so that you can clearly say what you mean and can communicate your needs without being whiney, aggressive, or argumentative.** Loads of assertiveness courses are available, and most workplaces offer them, too.

✔ **Stop comparing yourself to other people; you can never be like anyone else because you're original and unique.** On the other hand, do try to figure out how some people achieve things in their lives, and take a leaf out of their book; this can act as an inspiration.

✔ **Smile and never lose your sense of humor!**

✔ **Don't label yourself, or let other people label you, as being ill or different.** Feeling marginalized is enough to put anyone in a mental slump. You are you, and you're still able to reach goals and function very effectively in society, PCOS or no PCOS.

Emotional speak

Here are some statistics about what women feel about themselves, and this is not women with PCOS in particular:

✔ Sixty-four percent are plagued by unhappy thoughts about their weight and shape.

✔ Over 50 percent of women feel guilty about eating anything.

✔ Forty-one percent are in a constant battle between dieting and exercising, bingeing, and giving up trying.

So, having PCOS doesn't make it your unique prerogative to worry about such issues. Even so, the secret is to try to do something about your well-being without being totally hung up on it 24/7.

Stress: Know your limit

Some stress is good; it can motivate you to do things and give you a buzz about life. What you need to avoid is *distress,* which is what happens when stress gets pushed too far. Different people get stressed over different things, so situations that may make you berserk are what other people thrive on, and vice versa. However, coping with long-term ill health or uncertainty about how an illness changes or progresses is a recipe for stress in most people.

When you feel stressed you release a hormone called *cortisol.* A high level of this hormone has been associated with many of the same symptoms as PCOS such as:

- Increasing the likelihood that you're going to gain weight around your middle
- Increasing insulin resistance

Although acute and intense stress, such as becoming bereaved, can make you lose your appetite, *chronic stress* (when you're at a constant stressed-out state over a period of time) often leaves you reaching for food as a comforter.

The following sections offer tips you can try to limit the impact of stress.

Getting enough sleep

Different people need different amounts of sleep; the average is around seven hours of sleep a night, but if that still leaves you yawning and dopey the next day, up it by half an hour until you reach your ideal.

When you get into the swing of regular sleep, you find that you're better able to cope with the odd late night or sleepless night without it completely knocking you for a loop. You're also better able to cope with stress when you aren't tired. Don't forget that stress can tire you out in the first place and make you less likely to have a good night's sleep.

If you're stressed, a wind-down bedtime routine is essential, such as:

- Taking a bath
- Having a hot drink with milk (without caffeine!)
- Stopping work at least an hour before you go to bed

✔ Avoiding exercise at least an hour before bed

✔ Getting engrossed in a good book before you turn off the lights so that your mind isn't dwelling on the cares of the day — although this can backfire if the book's *too* good

Staying active

Do something physically active. Exercise reverses the negative effects of stress hormones. This doesn't have to be a formal exercise session — it may be a bout of spring cleaning or a brisk walk. Chapter 6 has some more ideas on how you can get more physically active.

Using relaxation techniques

Try some relaxation techniques. You can pick up CDs that take you through a relaxation exercise and show you how to breathe to help calm yourself. Many people tend to hyperventilate when stressed, which leaves them feeling dizzy, lightheaded, and with tingling in their hands and feet. Proper breathing can help you avoid doing this.

Keeping things in perspective

Put things in perspective by imagining your current situation and picturing the worst thing that could happen. Try to imagine yourself coping with that situation. Also, try to think how you're going to feel about your current situation in three months' time. These imagining techniques often help to put things in perspective and stop you from making mountains out of molehills.

Maintaining a balanced diet

Your body doesn't cope with stress very well if it feels deprived of food or fluid. Make sure you drink plenty of fluid during the day, and avoid caffeine if you're prone to stress or you don't sleep too well. Eating regular low-glycemic-index meals also helps your body to maintain a regular blood sugar level, which helps you cope better with stress.

Don't use props — such as caffeine or alcohol — to cope with stress. They may help you feel better in the short term, but payback time comes eventually and when that happens you feel ten times worse coping with caffeine- or alcohol-fueled sleep deprivation.

Strict dieting or eating an unbalanced diet will add extra stress to what your body already has to put up with. The best diet for de-stressing is to keep everything in moderation. If you need to cut the calories to reduce weight, the food you eat needs to be of good nutrient quality so that you don't lose out on your vitamins and minerals just because you're cutting back on the calories.

Have a nice cup of tea

Recent research from University College London shows that having a cup of tea after a stressful situation actually brings down the level of stress quickly. And it isn't just the act of sitting down and taking a break. The researchers took two groups of people and gave them both drinks that tasted the same, but one group had ordinary black tea in their drink, whereas the other group didn't. The researchers then subjected both groups to a stressful situation and gave them the drinks. Those who had the drink with the tea in it were found to recover from stress significantly more quickly than those who had the "dummy" drink. This was thought to be due to levels of the stress hormone cortisol being lowered more quickly in the tea drinkers.

Other stress busters

The list of potential stress-busters is limited only by your imagination! Here are a few more examples — they won't all suit you, but you may find that one of them is just the ticket!

- ✔ **Join a choir or take singing lessons.** The breathing exercises you learn and the act of actually singing helps to reduce stress levels.

- ✔ **Have a good laugh.** They often say laughter is a good medicine, and this saying contains some truth. Buy a few DVDs that are guaranteed to bring a smile to your face and dig them out when you feel stressed or gloomy.

- ✔ **Make plenty of time for yourself everyday.** Use it to do something you enjoy doing. Now and then, book yourself some indulgent time that doesn't center around food — maybe a massage or spa day, or just a long walk.

Are you feeling happy? Dealing with depression

Being down is not going to help you move on with your life; you may want to wallow in it all. Depression can be something that hovers over you like a dark cloud for an afternoon, or it can go on for months. If your depression is of the latter sort, get medical help. Although everyone hates taking medication, you may need some sort of antidepressant to help give you the impetus to sort out what's happening in your life.

Even short bouts of depression, if they happen often enough, can hinder your progress in tackling changes in your diet and lifestyle. Here are a few things to start doing — and a few to stop doing — in order to avoid bouts of depression:

✔ **Get enough sleep.** Lack of sleep can leave you feeling tired and unable to cope.

✔ **Don't take on too much.** This may be work, or helping out other people. You may need to cultivate some degree of selfishness in order to have the motivation to deal with your own challenges.

✔ **Don't drink too much alcohol.** Although your cares may seem like they float away for a while when you drink, they can come crashing back down on top of you worse than ever the next morning, leaving you feeling anxious and depressed.

✔ **Eat a good, balanced diet.** Have plenty of food variety to ensure that your body gets all the nutrients it needs. Being properly nourished and free from any nutritional deficiencies, however slight, maximizes your chances of not succumbing to depression.

A few promising studies have shown some benefit of eating plenty of oily fish or taking fish oil supplements to alleviate depression.

✔ **Don't isolate yourself.** If something is getting you down, try to talk it through with someone — a relative, your best friend, or even a trained counselor. Sometimes sharing worries with other people who know what you're going through can be good, so joining a PCOS network may help. With some of these networks, you may be able to share concerns online or attend regular meetings where you can meet with other sufferers.

✔ **Treat yourself from time to time.** Massage or aromatherapy sessions are good stress-busting treats.

Excuses, excuses

You'll always be able to find a reason not to adhere to your self-improvement plan. Life is so frantic and so full of snares that finding a good excuse for not doing something is easy. But at the end of the day you're only fooling yourself. You may have some really good reasons that genuinely make you incapable of applying yourself to any self-improvement plan, such as a major family trauma of some kind. However, if you're just experiencing chronic everyday stressors, you can still engage in some healthy eating and exercise. Plus, following a good diet and doing some exercise makes you better able to cope with everyday stress.

In addition to having too many other stressors in your life, Table 9-2 has some other common excuses as to why you're unable to adopt a healthy lifestyle — and why they just don't wash!

Table 9-2	Excuses and Solutions
Excuse	*Solution*
I don't like many healthy foods.	Keep trying lots of different fruits and veggies and less salty, fatty, and sugary foods, and after a few weeks, your taste buds will readjust.
I have to buy and cook different foods for the rest of the family, and then I get tempted to eat their foods.	Why inflict unhealthy food on the rest of the family? They can benefit from a healthier diet, too, so tell everyone it's a family effort.
Other people frequently cook for me, and when they've made something that shouldn't be part of my plan I don't like to refuse because it's rude.	If someone else cooks for you, tell him about your new regime and why following it is important. Kind cooks should understand.
Once I start eating, I can't stop!	Go for quality, not quantity. Don't let yourself get too hungry because this can trigger a binge. Eat several small low-glycemic-index meals so that blood sugars stay on an even keel.
Food is one of my great pleasures in life.	Then enjoy it, take time over it, ensure it's delicious, and again go for quality, not quantity. Also, work on some of those other pleasures of life, such as relaxing with a good book or going for a country walk.
Food calms me down and de-stresses me.	Somewhere in the past you started to use food as a comfort. This behavior can be broken by using other ways to calm yourself, such as yoga, a brisk walk, a hot bath with essential oils, or just some simple breathing exercises.
I can't exercise because I was no good at it in school.	Very few people, except for those picked for teams, enjoyed gym classes. Exercise is so much more than kickball, volleyball, and badminton. What about dancing, swimming, or even fencing? Find some activity you enjoy, and do it energetically!
I'm not fit enough to exercise.	Then start somewhere, and build up your fitness levels slowly. Everyone can get fitter, but if you don't use it, you lose it!
I don't have the time or money to exercise.	Fit in exercise around everyday activity. This approach may include cycling somewhere that involves a short journey rather than taking the car. This way you save money, too!

Talking about It

Keeping your worries and concerns all bottled up is not the way to move ahead. Different people can help in different ways; you can share some things with your mother, some with your girlfriends, and some with your partner, but other issues may require some professional advice.

Using your friends and family

Talk to friends and family, especially when you're feeling low and lacking in confidence. Surround yourself with people who have no ulterior motives. Being part of a friendship means that you confide in each other and share your worries and concerns. If you keep things to yourself all the time, people may think you're unapproachable and won't be willing to open up to you.

You can't always be the one who shares problems; to be a friendship, things have to work both ways. Sometimes offering a listening ear and support to your friend's problems can bring you out of your own slump or at least help to put yours in perspective.

Bringing in the professionals

Sometimes a problem is deep-rooted or doesn't seem to be resolving itself. Or you just can't bring yourself to talk it through with even your nearest and dearest. If this happens, it may be time to bring in a professional counselor. Your workplace may have a counseling service, or you may be able to get some advice from your doctor on which professional you need to see.

Fanaticism versus staying in control

When do you cross the line from staying in control to becoming a control freak or even a downright fanatic? You need to be able to stay in control but not make having control rule your life. When exerting reasonable control in your life becomes a fanatical behavior pattern, that line has been crossed. Eating disorders, for example, are the extreme end of trying to control food.

People who suffer from eating disorders spend their whole lives obsessing about their diets and foods. They impose very rigid food regimes on themselves as a way of trying to stay in control. And for the short term, they follow these regimes and feel powerful and confident. But they always set themselves impossible regimes to follow and soon slip up — which leads to a huge amount of self-loathing and stress. They try to get back on their strict regimes only to slip again and feel even worse, and so the pattern continues until ill health forces them, or those close to them, to seek help to break the cycle.

So, how can you avoid falling into the fanatics' trap? Here are some simple tips:

✔ **Don't set yourself up for failure by expecting too much of yourself.** Make your goal achievable and realistic. For example, losing 1 or 2 pounds a week is probably achievable, but 3 to 5 pounds isn't; getting to the gym three times a week may be achievable, but every day may not be.

✔ **Don't think of yourself as either on a diet or not on a diet.** Feeling that you're "on the wagon" is enough to make you want to jump off! Instead, just think of yourself as having chosen to eat a sensible diet in order to make yourself feel better. Don't forget that this new regime is probably something you're going to want to follow for life (with a few less calories if you're actively trying to lose weight). If you return to your old style of eating, you may end up back where you started in quite a short span of time.

✔ **Allow yourself to indulge occasionally.** This indulgence can be allowing yourself to slouch around in your pajamas all day rather than sticking to your exercise routine; or it may be to allow yourself an indulgent snack now and then. However, grant yourself that indulgence without seeing it as the beginning of the end. Know that you need to get straight back to your usual routine the next day, or the next meal.

✔ **Staying in control means being organized, but organization doesn't mean being inflexible if something unexpected crops up.** If too many things are happening that prevent you from following your chosen path — say, you find that you can never get to the gym — you may have to rethink your plan and perhaps clear some space for the gym by saying no to certain things. Or you may need to find a way to exercise outside the gym environment, closer to home.

Part III
Menstrual Cycles, Fertility, and Pregnancy

The 5th Wave   By Rich Tennant

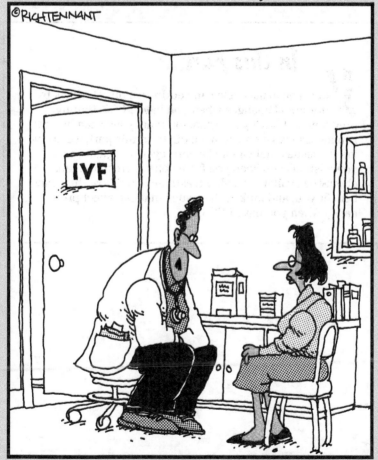

"In brief, we'll stimulate your ovaries with daily medications or hormones, perform an oocyte retrieval at the hospital, incubate the eggs in a Petri dish at the laboratory, and then sit back and let nature take its course."

In this part...

Your menstrual cycle can get thrown out of whack by hormonal changes when you have PCOS. Getting pregnant and having a normal pregnancy also can be challenging issues when you have PCOS. In this part, we examine the issues that can make your cycle irregular (or nonexistent) and keep you from getting pregnant, talk about the available fertility treatments and how they may benefit you, and look at the issues that can affect pregnancy when you have PCOS.

Chapter 10

Finding Your Periods: How PCOS Affects the Menstrual Cycle

In This Chapter

▶ Understanding how your reproductive system works

▶ Looking at the effects of hormonal changes

▶ Dealing with abnormal periods

▶ Recognizing potential problems resulting from not ovulating

*P*COS can have a huge impact on your hormones, which, in turn, have a huge impact on your menstrual cycle. Anything that impacts your menstrual cycle impacts your fertility. If it sounds like PCOS can really mess you up, reproductively speaking, you're right: It can. Not everyone will experience menstrual complications from PCOS, but it's good to know what can happen, so you can be on the lookout for potential problems.

Reviewing the Menstrual Cycle

When it comes to the menstrual cycle, it all starts with hormonal effects on the ovaries. And the ovaries are all about just one thing: producing an egg. As a quick review — or as a quick course if the mechanics behind the menstrual cycle have never interested you before — here's how things progress every month when you're having a normal menstrual period (see Figure 10-1):

1. **Gonadotropin-releasing hormone (GnRH), made in the *hypothalamus* (a structure in the middle of the brain that controls the endocrine system as well as the nervous system), stimulates LH and FSH production.**

2. **Follicle-stimulating hormone (FSH) is released by the pituitary gland (which is located at the base of the brain).**

   FSH stimulates the ovaries to start producing eggs. FSH levels at the start of a menstrual cycle normally are less than 10 mIU/mL or 11 mIU/mL.

3. **Between 10 and 15 follicles begin to grow in the ovaries, each in its own fluid-filled sac.**

   Only one follicle normally continues to grow to maturity. Estrogen is released by the growing follicle. Estrogen levels rise as the follicle matures.

   There are several different types of estrogen, including estradiol (the main form of estrogen), estrone, and estriol. Estradiol levels usually fall between 10 pg/mL and less than 80 pg/mL at the start of a menstrual cycle.

4. **As estrogen is released, FSH is suppressed. As the egg nears maturity, luteinizing hormone (LH) is released from the pituitary.**

   LH is necessary for egg development, estrogen production, and egg release from the ovaries. At the start of the cycle, LH is usually around 5 mIU/mL, but it rises to 40 mIU/mL or so just before ovulation in a normal menstrual cycle.

5. **LH matures the egg and allows it to burst out of the follicle, a process called *ovulation*. LH also causes enzyme changes in the follicle so that the follicle begins to produce progesterone.**

6. **The follicle collapses and becomes the *corpus luteum* (the remnant of the follicle that held the developing egg), and progesterone readies the uterine lining for implantation.**

   Pre-ovulation levels of progesterone are low, less than 1.5 ng/mL. Progesterone levels normally rise to or more after ovulation. During pregnancy, the placenta takes over progesterone production.

7. **FSH production stops, so no more eggs are matured.**

8. **If no pregnancy occurs, the corpus luteum degenerates and stops producing progesterone.**

   The uterine lining breaks down and your period starts.

As you can see, several hormones — estrogen, progesterone, FSH, GnRH, and LH — play a part in the monthly production of an egg, and they all, like actors in a play, interact with each other. An imbalance in one hormone, like one bad actor in a play, can throw off the whole production. Like actors responding to each other's lines, hormones respond to one another in a feedback loop that allows the secretion of one hormone to reduce production of another.

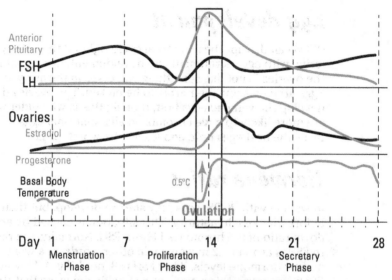

Figure 10-1: The menstrual cycle involves a complex interplay between hormones.

Hormones not directly involved with the menstrual cycle but that can impact its functioning include the following:

- ✔ **Insulin:** Women with PCOS often have higher-than-normal levels of insulin, which is released in response to glucose in the bloodstream. (See Chapter 3 for more about the important part insulin plays in PCOS.) Increased insulin levels can trigger increased androgen production from the ovaries. (*Androgens* are male hormones that cause many of the symptoms of PCOS.)

- ✔ **Prolactin:** Prolactin, produced by the pituitary gland, is normally suppressed except during pregnancy and lactation. Because prolactin inhibits GnRH, high prolactin levels can stop follicular production in the ovaries, causing *anovulation* (lack of ovulation) and *amenorrhea* (lack of menstrual periods).

Identifying the Effects of Hormone Changes in PCOS

The hormonal changes that occur in PCOS affect every aspect of the menstrual cycle, from how often menstruation occurs to how often you ovulate and how well your eggs develop. Good eggs are a pregnancy prerequisite!

This section discusses the way hormones can affect your cycle and the consequences that accompany these changes.

Egg development

PCOS can disrupt the menstrual cycle right off the bat, by interfering with egg recruitment and development. Egg recruitment in the ovaries is not like something you'd see in the army, of course. Eggs aren't waving their arms to be picked. The ovaries do try to develop the winning eggs first, though; this is why older women are more likely to have chromosomally abnormal eggs — nature takes the best eggs first, and leaves the worst for last.

Hormone ratios

In women with PCOS, eggs may start to develop, but then fizzle out before they reach maturity. This situation is caused by an upside-down ratio of the hormones LH and FSH. Normally, the ratio of LH to FSH is around 1:2 in women. In other words, in a woman with normal hormone levels, if her FSH is 8, her LH is 4. In women with PCOS, however, this ratio is often upside-down, so that the level of LH is two or three times higher than the level of FSH. Not all women with PCOS have an abnormal LH:FSH ratio — in fact, fewer than 50 percent do, and only around 20 percent of women with PCOS have an inverted ratio as high as 3:1.

An abnormal LH:FSH ratio leads to problems such as an overproduction of androgens. Androgens are produced in the ovaries, so if the ovaries are busy producing androgens, it doesn't produce enough estrogen to keep the growing follicle going. High levels of insulin also can contribute to androgen production.

Although this upside-down ratio doesn't affect all women with PCOS, when it does, it interferes with egg development. An egg may start to develop when stimulated by FSH, but the higher LH levels stop the development. The egg doesn't grow, but it also doesn't release, so no ovulation occurs.

Lack of ovulation

When the growing follicle doesn't release the egg inside, it develops into a cyst. Women with PCOS often have multiple pearly cysts inside each ovary (see Figure 10-2), which make the ovary larger than normal. (Although 90 percent of women with PCOS have enlarged ovaries, 25 percent or so of women *without* PCOS have enlarged ovaries, too.)

Cysts continue to produce small amounts of estrogen, which stimulate the uterine lining. Without the corpus luteum remnant from the ovulated follicle, no progesterone is produced. The lining doesn't get a signal to break down, so it keeps thickening.

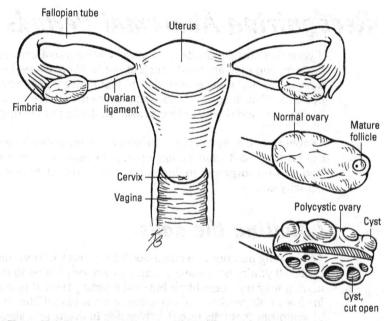

Figure 10-2: The ovaries in women with PCOS contain many small cysts.

If you have a pelvic ultrasound done, your ovaries will appear larger than normal, with 10 to 15 small cysts (usually less than 10 mm in size) in each ovary. Most of the cysts in the ovaries will be on the surface rather than in the center of the ovaries.

Menstrual changes

The thicker-than-normal lining produced by constant estrogen stimulation (see the preceding section) will eventually break down, but it may take several months. This is why many women with PCOS have irregular menstrual cycles.

When menstrual periods do occur, they're often very heavy, because the lining has become much thicker than normal. Signs of a heavier-than-normal period include the following:

✔ Menstrual flow that lasts more than seven days

✔ Saturating a pad or tampon in less than an hour for several hours in a row

✔ Passing clots

✔ Severe cramping

Recognizing Abnormal Periods

If your menstrual periods have always fallen into a certain irregular pattern, you may not think much about it. Many women with PCOS have never had regular periods and just figure that their abnormal cycles are "normal" for them. Many women also don't realize that having a period doesn't always mean that you're ovulating.

Keeping track of your cycles for several months can help your doctor figure out what's going on in your reproductive organs. You may be surprised to find out just how irregular your periods actually are.

Counting the days

An amazing number of women don't keep track of their menstrual cycles. If you're not sexually active or actively trying to get pregnant, it may not seem like a big deal if your period doesn't come for five or six weeks — or even five or six months! This is the sort of symptom that falls into the "blessing in disguise" category for some women.

However, nearly all normal menstrual cycles fall into the 24- to 34-day range; if yours don't, you should find out why, especially if you're planning on getting pregnant in the future. If you're having what seem like very light periods every few weeks, you may be experiencing *breakthrough bleeding,* which occurs when a very thick lining sheds a little at a time.

Most of the time, PCOS causes abnormally long rather than short cycles. If your menstrual cycles come more frequently than every 24 days, you may be dealing with other problems related to a high FSH level.

Tracking the flow

Very heavy, irregular periods are one of the hallmarks of PCOS, but you could also experience periods that are really just dribbles and drabs — a few spots here, a few there. This is more likely to be the effect of small bits of the uterine lining shedding than an actual menstrual period.

Get a calendar large enough to write in and keep track of exactly what you experience, flow-wise, for several months. Believe it or not, it's difficult to remember how often you had a little bleeding; it's hard enough to remember when your last period was, much less the last six months' worth!

Write down when the bleeding started, how long it lasted and how heavy it was. Because this is the sort of information you may not want on your kitchen calendar for the whole world to see, buy a calendar you can tuck in your purse or your lingerie drawer.

When You Don't Ovulate

As many as 75 percent of women who don't ovulate at all, a condition called *anovulation,* or ovulate only occasionally, a condition called *oligo-ovulation,* have PCOS. Anovulation or oligo-ovulation are classic signs of PCOS and defining characteristics for being diagnosed with the disorder. Anovulation can cause your uterine lining to become too thick, which is a risk factor for uterine cancer and also can make it impossible to get pregnant.

How to determine whether you're ovulating

It's not always that easy to recognize when you're not ovulating. Some women get what appear to be fairly regular periods even though they're not producing an egg, or not releasing an egg that starts to develop.

There are some clues that you're not ovulating regularly or at all. Suspect that you're not ovulating if:

- ✓ Your periods don't fall into any sort of pattern.

- ✓ You never experience *mittelshmerz,* the pain felt by as many as 20 percent of women when an egg releases from the follicle.

- ✓ You don't suffer from premenstrual syndrome, with symptoms such as mood swings or stomach cramps in the few days before your period starts.

- ✓ You don't experience a rise in your body temperature around two weeks before the start of your period. A slight drop, followed by a rise in basal body temperature taken first thing in the morning, usually indicates ovulation (see the nearby sidebar).

- ✓ You don't notice a change in cervical mucus at any point during your cycle. Normally, around the time of ovulation, cervical mucus becomes thinner, stretchy, more alkaline, and more copious to give sperm a more hospitable environment.

Checking for ovulation by taking your basal body temperature

One of the oldest time-honored methods of determining whether you're ovulating is use of the basal body temperature. To do this, you need a thermometer that's easy to read and that registers small increments. A digital thermometer, a thermometer that you use in your ear, or a glass thermometer with more precise markings that registers changes to one-tenth of a degree is ideal.

Take your temperature every morning before you even sit up. Don't go to the bathroom, drink, smoke, or do anything else that might raise your temperature. Yes, that includes having sex!

Record your temperature daily. Some thermometers save the last reading so you can check it later if you forget. A glass thermometer will show the last reading until you shake it down.

Watch for a dip. Right before ovulation, your temperature will drop slightly, maybe by as little as two-tenths of a degree.

Watch for a rise of ½ to 1 degree after ovulation. Progesterone raises your body temperature, so if you produced a good follicle and ovulated, the corpus luteum will make progesterone.

If you're actively trying to pinpoint ovulation to get pregnant, one telltale sign may come from using ovulation prediction kits (OPKs). Sold over-the-counter, these "pee on a stick" tests use urine to determine when ovulation is about to occur.

Since OPKs test LH levels, which rise around 24 to 48 hours before ovulation, you may never get a positive reading. It's also possible that you may have a high reading all the time, if your LH levels, which are higher than normal in women with PCOS, are high enough to trigger the positive reading on the test.

Women with PCOS may start to develop an egg that doesn't complete its development. If you have a weak LH surge before ovulation, you may have a positive OPK, because the test doesn't give exact numbers — it's a qualitative, yes-or-no test, not a quantitative test, which gives an exact reading. But if the surge is weak, the egg won't mature and release properly.

 One way to be sure you don't have a permanently high LH is to test with OPKs at various times of the month. You can't always be ovulating, so you may have an abnormally high LH and aren't ovulating. Follow up with a blood test to check your LH levels.

Blood tests are a definitive way to tell whether you're ovulating. A single blood test won't give you the answers you need; you'll need to test at several times, including

- ✔ The start of the month to establish baseline numbers.

- ✔ A week or so after your period starts, to see if your estrogen levels are rising.

- ✔ Around mid-cycle, to check for an LH surge.

- ✔ After the time of suspected ovulation, to see if progesterone levels rise appropriately. If there's no corpus luteum because no egg was released, progesterone levels won't rise.

Uterine lining buildup

If you're not trying to get pregnant, not having periods may seem like a blessing in disguise. But not having periods can cause problems with your uterine lining, also called the *endometrium*.

Although you can't tell, your lining may be getting thicker under the influence of estrogen. You may not be producing enough estrogen from the ovaries to trigger egg development, but you may be producing enough to signal your uterus that it should be thickening.

Checking up on your lining

It's easy to find out what's happening inside your uterus — all you need is a pelvic ultrasound. A pelvic ultrasound can be done abdominally or vaginally. For an abdominal test, you'll need to have a full bladder. A vaginal ultrasound gives a clearer picture, particularly if you're overweight.

During an ultrasound, the thickness of your uterine lining can be measured. A normal lining

- ✔ Measures around 3 mm at day two or three of your menstrual cycle

- ✔ Increases to between 8 mm and 13 mm, optimally, by the middle of the menstrual cycle

Problems with a thick lining

A lining that doesn't shed obviously keeps getting thicker. Although you can't feel this, you may experience breakthrough bleeding with a thick lining. But the real risks of an abnormally thick uterine lining, also called *endometrial hyperplasia,* involve the possibility of cancer developing in the endometrium.

Around 95 percent of all uterine cancers arise in the lining and are called *adenocarcinomas*. Age, obesity, and a history of unopposed estrogen influence on the uterus all increase the risk of uterine adenocarcinoma.

Unopposed estrogen simply means that the uterus gets estrogen stimulation without progesterone to balance it; this is why birth control pills often contain both estrogen and progesterone. When progesterone levels drop, the uterine lining breaks down and a period begins.

The most common sign of uterine cancer is abnormal bleeding, but most women with PCOS who have abnormal bleeding do not have cancer. If your doctor is concerned about the thickness of your endometrium, a simple biopsy of the lining, which removes a small piece to be examined under a microscope for signs of cancer, can set your mind at ease.

Pregnancy problems

PCOS is a common cause of infertility. Most of the time, infertility in women with PCOS is related to anovulation, because it's not possible to get pregnant if you're not producing or releasing an egg.

Getting diagnosed

For many women, an inability to get pregnant is the first real sign that they have PCOS. This isn't surprising when you consider that as many as 25 percent of women don't realize they have polycystic ovaries because no one has ever put their symptoms together.

Many women take oral contraceptives up until the time they want to get pregnant, and oral contraceptives, which are often given as a treatment for PCOS, can mask the symptoms of the disorder. Women who have taken oral contraceptives since they were in their teens may never have developed the more obvious signs of PCOS such as *hirsutism* (abnormal hair growth on the face, back, or chest).

When women who have been taking the pill long-term stop taking it, they may have more success getting pregnant immediately off the pill, which has suppressed their androgen levels. If they wait several months after stopping the pill, though, they may find that their periods have stopped.

Infertility is defined as the absence of pregnancy in a couple actively trying to get pregnant for a period of six months to one year. If you know you have PCOS and you aren't sure you're ovulating, there's no reason to wait six months to see your gynecologist or a fertility specialist.

Establishing the cause

Your doctor can determine whether you're ovulating simply by checking your blood work. A pelvic ultrasound helps confirm the presence of polycystic ovaries.

Multiple factors often contribute to infertility — there may be more than one reason why you're not getting pregnant, including problems with your partner. Although it's common to focus on the obvious cause, in as many as 10 percent to 20 percent of infertility cases, both partners have issues contributing to the problem. A simple semen analysis can establish that you have good sperm to work with, when you do start ovulating.

Here's a checklist of blood tests your doctor may want to run, in addition to estradiol, LH, FSH, and progesterone levels; most of the following tests are done at the start of a menstrual cycle on day two or three:

- ✔ **Total and free testosterone:** All women have some testosterone, just as all men have some estrogen. Both the total testosterone level and the amount of active, unbound testosterone, called *free testosterone,* are checked. The normal total testosterone range is between 6 ng/dL and 86 ng/dL, while the normal level of free testosterone ranges from 0.7 pg/mL to 3.6 pg/mL. Women with PCOS often have higher-than-normal levels of both. A total testosterone level of 50 is considered somewhat elevated.

- ✔ **Dehydroepiandrosterone (DHEA):** DHEA is another type of male hormone also found in smaller amounts in women. The normal range in women is 35 ug/dL to 430 ug/dL, but levels peak when you're in your 20s and decrease as you get older. Women with PCOS may have higher-than-normal levels of DHEA.

- ✔ **Glucose:** Checking your fasting glucose levels to make sure you don't have diabetes or pre-diabetes before trying to get pregnant is a good idea if you have PCOS. Your fasting blood glucose level should be less than 100 mg/dL; a level between 100 and 125 indicated pre-diabetes and the strong possibility of developing diabetes in the future.

- ✔ **Insulin:** Higher than normal levels of insulin are a common sign of insulin resistance. A fasting insulin level should be below 10 IU/mL; levels between 10 IU/mL and 30 IU/mL indicate insulin resistance, with higher levels usually indicating more insulin resistance.

- ✔ **Sex hormone binding globulin (SHBG):** SHBG is a glycoprotein that binds to estrogen and testosterone. Low levels of SHBG are typical of PCOS. Normal levels range between 18 nmol/L and 114 nmol/L at the start of the menstrual cycle.

Getting started on getting pregnant

There's nothing wrong with trying on your own for a while if you want to, but follow these guidelines to maximize your chances of success:

- **Check for ovulation.** See "How to determine whether you're ovulating," earlier in this chapter, for tips on making sure you're actually ovulating.

- **Pay attention to timing.** Timing is everything in getting pregnant. You can't get pregnant any old time of the month, because sperm don't live forever, not even really good ones. You need to have sex around the time of ovulation so that an egg is available once the sperm reach their destination. Do this by one of these methods:

    • **Have sex every other day throughout the cycle.** Sperm live around three days, so this method guarantees that fresh sperm will be available whenever the egg rolls down the hatch.

    • **Have sex around the time of ovulation, planning for the day before and the day of ovulation to cover your bases.** This requires being really attuned to your cycle and can put extra stress — never a good thing when trying to get pregnant, for either of you — on a potentially already stressful situation.

Making sure you have sex on the big "O" day may seem all-consuming to you, but try not to relay your anxieties to your partner — after all, he's the one who has to "perform" to bring this production to a close. This is where the every-other-day method can come in handy. There's no additional "big day" pressure — you don't even have to tell him when the day is, until after the performance! Knowing that if he can't come through, all is lost is no way to improve a man's sexual ability.

Chapter 11

Getting Pregnant: Infertility Treatments for PCOS

- -

In This Chapter

▶ Getting ready to get pregnant

▶ Talking to your doctor when you're ready to start trying

▶ Upping your efforts when pregnancy doesn't come easily

▶ Seeing a fertility specialist

▶ Dealing with disappointment

- -

*I*nfertility is, sad to say, a common occurrence in women with PCOS. As many as 20 percent of all cases of infertility involve PCOS. Between 90 percent and 95 percent of women who attend fertility clinics due to lack of ovulation are believed to be PCOS sufferers. That doesn't mean, however, that you can't get pregnant! Statistics also show that as many as 70 percent of women with PCOS start ovulating after simple treatment and, of those, around 30 percent get pregnant within the next three months.

So, although fertility treatment can involve complex and expensive treatment, many women with PCOS do get pregnant fairly easily with minimal treatment.

When pregnancy doesn't happen overnight — or even over a couple months — you have several choices. One is to keep trying and hope that nature will eventually take its course. The other is to ratchet up your efforts and look at anything and everything that could be standing between you and a baby. Often, that means seeing a fertility specialist and going through fertility treatments. In this chapter, we tell you what to expect and how to cope with the stresses of infertility.

Taking Some Initial Steps on Your Own

It can be discouraging to think that PCOS can have such a negative effect on what most people consider an inalienable right — the right to have children when you want them. But you're not hopeless in the fight against infertility when you have PCOS; in fact, some of the simplest measures, like losing weight, can have the biggest effects. In this section, we tell you steps you can take when you're trying to get pregnant with PCOS.

Losing weight

If nothing else has given you the impetus to lose weight, the desire to get pregnant might. Losing weight before you even try to get pregnant is ideal.

Here's how extra weight affects your chances of getting pregnant: Increased weight leads to the muscles becoming resistant to the effects of insulin. More insulin is produced in order to have the same desired effect on the muscles. You end up with a condition called *hyperinsulinemia,* where high levels of insulin are circulating in your blood. The high insulin levels affect other hormones in the body, and your ovaries overproduce testosterone. Too much testosterone leads to abnormal production of the hormones LH and FSH (see Chapter 10 for more on these hormones). Abnormal production of LH and FSH causes the ovaries to underproduce estrogen and progesterone and continue to overproduce testosterone. The result is that the follicles in the ovary (which contain your eggs) don't reach maturity. This means that no egg is released. Without an egg being released, you can't get pregnant.

Here's why losing weight is important if you're dealing with infertility:

- ✔ **Even a small weight loss improves your chances of getting pregnant.** You don't need to be a size 2 — in fact, it's better not to be that thin, because very thin women often don't ovulate either. Even adjusting your body weight downward by around 10 percent can increase your odds of getting pregnant by getting ovulation going again.

- ✔ **You're less likely to have complications in pregnancy.** Overweight women have an increased risk of nearly every pregnancy complication, from gestational diabetes and hypertension to preterm delivery and Cesarean section. Because PCOS also increases your odds of some of these pregnancy complications, losing weight will reduce your risks on both fronts.

✔ **In vitro fertilization (IVF) procedures will be easier.** If you get this far down the road, doing an egg retrieval (see the section "Moving On to a Fertility Specialist," later in this chapter) will be much simpler if you lose some weight. Visualizing or reaching the ovaries during egg retrieval is sometime difficult in women who are considerably overweight.

In your zeal to get pregnant, don't go on a crash diet. Crash diets can slow your metabolism and increase your risk of developing gallbladder problems. Follow the low-GI diet recommended in Chapter 4. *Remember:* Slow and steady is the healthiest way to lose weight.

You may find you don't need any further fertility help after losing a small amount of weight — a rather astounding 70 percent of women whose infertility is related to being overweight or underweight get pregnant spontaneously when they reach a normal weight!

Quitting smoking

Quit smoking immediately — both of you. Women who smoke are 50 percent more likely to miscarry and two to four times more likely to have an ectopic pregnancy, which develops in the Fallopian tubes. Smokers also have a higher percentage of abnormal eggs. Men who smoke are more likely to have a lower than normal sperm count. And secondhand smoke isn't good for anyone — pregnant or not pregnant.

Supplementing with vitamins

While you're thinking about diet, also give some thought to dietary supplements. All women who are trying to get pregnant should take at least 400 micrograms of folic acid per day, to decrease the risk of neural tube defects, which include *spina bifida* (an abnormal opening in the spine) and *anencephaly* (the absence of a large part of the brain and skull). Neural tube defects occur very early in pregnancy, so don't wait until you're pregnant to take this important nutrient!

Taking high-dose supplements isn't necessary and may even be harmful. Multivitamin and mineral supplements designed especially for pregnancy are usually okay, but make sure that they don't provide huge doses of any one nutrient. A recent study published in the respected medical journal *The Lancet* showed that high doses of vitamins C and E taken during pregnancy actually increase the risk of having a baby with a low birth weight. The researchers, however, confirmed that doses of these antioxidant vitamins taken in the amounts found in a multivitamin supplement didn't pose a threat.

If you're anemic, as often happens if you've had very heavy periods, your doctor may prescribe iron supplements in addition to the iron in your prenatal vitamin.

Ask your doctor before taking any supplements.

Limiting your alcohol consumption

Having more than three drinks per day can make your menstrual cycles irregular and decrease your chances of getting pregnant, so quit or drink only moderately — which, for women, means no more than one drink per day — when you're trying to get pregnant.

 Quit drinking completely as soon as you get pregnant. Alcohol increases your risk of miscarriage and can cause fetal alcohol syndrome, which causes behavioral and learning problems along with facial malformations.

Being prudent with prescription drugs

Ask your doctor about any potential side effects from the prescription drugs you take as you're trying to get pregnant. And, although it should go without saying, avoid *all* illegal drugs.

Putting a cap on caffeine

To be on the safe side, experts recommend that women who are pregnant, or planning to become pregnant, limit their caffeine intake to about 300 mg of caffeine per day, which is around four cups of coffee. Don't forget that other drinks, such as colas and teas, also contain caffeine!

Seeing Your Doctor

Hopefully, you're already working with your gynecologist and potential obstetrician, even before you start trying to get pregnant. Having an OB-GYN you like and trust helps make the process of trying to get pregnant if not easier than at least more comfortable.

When you're ready to start trying to get pregnant, schedule an appointment with your gynecologist to talk about your chances. Every woman with PCOS is different. Here are some of the issues that may factor into your chances of success:

- ✔ **Your age:** Your chances for pregnancy decrease with age. Over age 40, fertility rates falls off considerably, and over 45, they're just slightly over nonexistent — but it does happen!

- ✔ **Your reproductive organs:** The condition of your uterus, Fallopian tubes, and ovaries can greatly impact your odds of pregnancy without assisted reproductive technology. (See the next section for more on the tests that are done to evaluate your reproductive organs.)

> ✔ **Your partner's sperm:** Although you may hardly believe that life could be so cruel as to hand you lousy sperm along with PCOS, it does happen and there are treatments. (See "Sending the boys out for a checkup," later in this chapter.)

Ratcheting Up Your Efforts

If you're having trouble getting pregnant, it's time to schedule a few tests. Your regular gynecologist can do these, in most cases.

Having a hysterosalpingo . . . what?

Also known as the dye test or an HSG, the nearly unpronounceable hysterosalpingogram evaluates the interior of your uterus and Fallopian tubes. An HSG is usually done in the first half of the menstrual cycle, to avoid disrupting a potential pregnancy. Dye is injected through the cervix and then tracked on X-ray as it traverses the uterus and Fallopian tubes.

An HSG is somewhat uncomfortable; you lie on your back while the dye is injected. Some women feel cramping, which is caused by the instruments as well as the distention of the uterus. You may feel shoulder pain as the dye goes through the tubes, especially if there's a blockage in the tubes.

When to seek help getting pregnant

Deciding when it's time to seek professional help depends on several factors, including your age as well as how patient you are. Some women have the patience to try for a full year without seeking medical advice; others want to see a specialist if they're not pregnant within ten minutes after deciding to try. Only you know your own patience level.

If you're under age 35 and have PCOS but have regular menstrual cycles, trying for six months is reasonable. If you're not having menstrual periods, you're not going to get pregnant, no matter how long you try, so see your doctor as soon as you decide it's time to have a baby, if not before.

Women who are over age 40 often have issues getting pregnant even if they don't have PCOS, so consider seeing your doctor even before trying to get pregnant. Irregular periods in your 40s could mean PCOS or the start of perimenopause; your doctor can help you sort out exactly what's going on.

An HSG can diagnose a number of abnormalities that could be interfering with pregnancy:

- ✔ **Uterine fibroids:** These extremely common benign growths occur in around 75 percent of all women. Black women are especially likely to have fibroids. Most fibroids don't have any impact on getting pregnant, but if they're located in certain places — intruding into the endometrial cavity, for instance — they may interfere with embryo implantation.

- ✔ **Polyps:** Polyps are small, fleshy outgrowths of tissue that also can interfere with pregnancy implantation. Polyps can be easily removed during a minor procedure called a *hysteroscopy.*

- ✔ **Endometriosis:** If your Fallopian tubes have been damaged over the years by endometriosis or by sexually transmitted diseases such as chlamydia, the sperm may not be able to get to the egg or an embryo may have trouble getting from the ovary to the uterus.

Blocked or infected Fallopian tubes are best treated with IVF. In some cases, if the tubes have a chronic infection known as *hydrosalpinx,* your doctor may even suggest removing them altogether, because toxins in the tube can affect the uterine environment and interfere with implantation.

For more on endometriosis, check out *Endometriosis For Dummies,* by Joseph W. Krotec, MD, and Sharon Perkins, RN (Wiley).

Other ways to look inside

An HSG isn't the only way to get a look around the inside of the uterus. In fact, your doctor can look directly inside by doing a hysteroscopy and may even be able to remove polyps or fibroids at the same time. A simpler test called a *sonohysterogram* gives similar results to an HSG except that it doesn't evaluate the Fallopian tubes.

Having a hysteroscopy

In a hysteroscopy, your doctor will distend the uterus with carbon dioxide and then use a lighted scope to look directly into the uterus. Polyps and small fibroids as well as adhesions can be removed during an operative hysteroscopy, which is done under a nerve block or possibly an epidural or general anesthesia, depending on how much work needs to be done.

Seeing with a sonohysterogram

A sonohysterogram is similar to an HSG except that saline instead of dye is injected. Instead of following the dye via X-ray, ultrasound is used. Abnormalities in the uterus such as fibroids, adhesions, and polyps can be seen in a sonohysterogram. This test is normally done in the doctor's office without medication.

Looking laparoscopically

A laparoscopy is a surgical procedure normally done through small incision that allows placement of instruments and a lighted scope. Laparoscopy requires anesthesia and is done in the hospital or in a same-day surgical center. Laparoscopy is used to remove endometriosis or to remove damaged Fallopian tubes.

The doctor inflates your abdomen with carbon dioxide, which may cause shoulder pain for a day. The incisions also may cause pain for several days. The recovery period is normally less than a week for laparoscopy.

Sending the boys out for a checkup

Your partner may balk at doing a semen analysis, for reasons ranging from performance anxiety to fear of finding out his boys have issues. But we can't stress enough that just because you have one fertility issue doesn't mean you don't have two — or more. Don't pin all your fertility blame on PCOS without checking out other possibilities.

Nearly all sperm deficiencies can be overcome with good lab work in the fertility lab, so don't worry if the report doesn't list glowing numbers. Sperm can be concentrated in the lab to give a higher yield, so to speak. During IVF, the lab tech can pick out the prettiest sperm of the bunch and inject it directly into an egg, a procedure called *intracycloplasmic sperm injection* (ICSI). (See "Moving On to a Fertility Specialist," later in this chapter, for more on sperm techniques.)

Here's what the lab wants to see when looking at the little swimmers:

- ✔ **Number:** Nature is incredibly wasteful with sperm, it would seem; an acceptable sperm count contains 20 million sperm per milliliter, or 40 million per ejaculate! However, many sperm are abnormal and others get lost in crevasses, go the wrong way, or otherwise shoot themselves in the proverbial foot on the way to the egg. It also takes a collective effort of many sperm to crack through the egg. You ideally need every one of those 20 million.

- ✔ **Movement:** Sperm have someplace to go, and although the initial propulsion can move them into the uterus through the cervix, they may still have the equivalent of a few miles ahead of them to reach the egg. Around 40 percent of the sperm should move forward rather than in circles or not at all.

✔ **Morphology:** Good sperm are better looking, at least in the lab tech's eyes. Sperm should conform to normal standards of having a shaped head of a standard size and one normal-size tail. Around 30 percent of sperm should have normal morphology in order to bring a smile to the lab tech's face, if the lab uses the WHO criteria. If they use the stricter Kruger morphology to rate sperm, 14 percent should be normal.

Kruger strict morphology uses a more stringent classification system that grades only perfect sperm as normal. Many fertility clinics use Kruger strict morphology criteria.

Trying a little Clomid

Clomid is like the aspirin of the fertility world; the first thing your gynecologist may tell you if you're not getting pregnant is to "Take two Clomid and call me if you're not pregnant in a few months."

Actually, it's not quite that simple, and if you have PCOS, it's even less simple, because Clomid can cause multiple births, especially in people with PCOS.

How Clomid works

Clomiphene citrate is a pill that fools your body into thinking it's not making enough estrogen. The following sequence of events hopefully leads to ovulation after you take Clomid:

1. **The hypothalamus releases gonadotropin-releasing hormone (GnRH).**

    Yes, everything in fertility does seem to have long, incomprehensible names.

2. **The release of GnRH stimulates the release of FSH.**

    See Chapter 10 for a quick review of reproductive hormones.

3. **FSH stimulates the ovary to produce an egg.**

4. **The ovary responds and an egg starts to develop.**

You take Clomid for five days, normally, starting between days two and four of the menstrual cycle — physicians have different ideas about what works best. Your doctor may start with just one 50 mg tablet per day and move you up to two if you don't get pregnant within a few months.

What your other half can do

In addition to being supportive, your partner can take some positive steps (along with avoiding some things) to maximize the chance of pregnancy.

Drugs (medicinal as well as recreational), alcohol, and cigarettes all take their toll on sperm quality. If your partner works with certain chemicals, he should check whether they're known to have an effect on sperm quality, too.

Here's a list of some other factors that can have an effect on sperm quality as well as reduce male fertility:

✓ **Fever:** Flu, or even a severe cold, can cause a high fever, which adversely affects sperm production and quality. These subsequent temporary drops usually recover over a few weeks, which is why you should not make decisions based on a single semen sample.

✓ **Diabetes:** In the long term, diabetes can cause problems with erection and ejaculation.

✓ **High blood pressure:** High blood pressure can cause problems with erection, either directly or as a side effect of medication.

✓ **Arterial disease:** Arterial disease can cause problems with erection. This can be due to generalized hardening of the arteries, in the penis as well as the heart, or to drugs used in the treatment of heart problems.

✓ **Neurological disorders:** Disorders such as multiple sclerosis, spinal injury, or stroke all can cause problems with erection and ejaculation.

✓ **Kidney disease:** Kidney disease can result in a buildup of waste products in the body, adversely affecting sperm quality and fertility. It also can cause erection problems.

✓ **Cancer:** Cancer can affect the genital tract or endocrine (hormone-producing) system and may directly reduce fertility. Otherwise, drugs and radiation used to treat cancer may severely reduce sperm production or even stop it altogether. Freezing sperm before chemotherapy is a good option.

✓ **Alcoholism:** Alcohol is toxic to sperm, and overuse of alcohol can reduce sperm quality and fertility.

✓ **Stress:** Stress causes several hormonal changes in the body that can affect fertility.

Clocking the effects

Although many doctors don't monitor women taking Clomid, it may be a good idea to get an ultrasound and bloodwork midcycle while you're on Clomid if you have PCOS. Between 5 percent and 10 percent of all Clomid pregnancies produce twins, while 1 in 400 produces triplets and 1 in 800 produces quadruplets. Multiple births are more likely to happen if you have PCOS; a little stimulation may turn your ovaries into overachievers.

Unless you want to end up with your own reality show someday, you may choose not to try to get pregnant in a month when you make 10 or 12 eggs. In fact, many fertility specialists will refuse to do an intrauterine insemination in these cases.

Dealing with the side effects

Because your body thinks you don't have enough estrogen, you may experience menopause-like symptoms, such as hot flashes, headaches, blurred vision, or nausea, when taking Clomid. Clomid also can interfere with cervical mucus production, which can make it difficult for sperm to get through the cervix.

Adding a little extra

If your cervical mucus production has been decimated by Clomid or if you're dealing with sperm issues on top of everything else, doing an intrauterine insemination (IUI) not only will ensure that the sperm are where they should be, but also will give them a leg up on going the rest of the way. (See "Moving On to a Fertility Specialist" for more on IUIs.)

Maybe a little metformin

Metformin is a medication that lowers blood glucose levels by improving insulin resistance. Metformin was developed and tested for treatment of type 2 diabetes and is still used for that purpose. However, metformin also is used to decrease insulin resistance in women with PCOS. (See Chapter 7 for the whole story on metformin.)

Because metformin reduces insulin resistance, it may help reverse the whole insulin resistance cascade described in the "Losing weight for pregnancy" section, earlier in this chapter. If you haven't been on metformin up to this point, starting it now may help you start ovulating again so you can get pregnant.

Moving On to a Fertility Specialist

If relatively simple measures like a few rounds of Clomid don't result in pregnancy, it may be time to move up to the big guns — assisted reproductive technology. Your regular gynecologist will probably bow out of the picture at this point, hopefully to be reintroduced when you get pregnant in a few months.

Fertility specialists are often, but not always, reproductive endocrinologists — gynecologists who've had additional training to become certified in infertility and other issues related to the reproductive and endocrine systems.

Finding a specialist

Fertility specialists are usually not shy about advertising their specialty; many advertise in parenting or family-oriented magazines or in newspapers. The Internet is an easy way to search for fertility specialists near you. Although a fertility specialist who focuses on PCOS would be nice, it isn't necessary — all fertility specialists deal with a large number of women with PCOS.

Finding a specialist is easy, but finding one you want to work with can be more complicated. To make it easier, consider these issues:

- ✔ **Insurance:** Fertility treatment is expensive. Start first with your insurance company, and find out who takes your insurance.

- ✔ **Proximity:** Fertility treatment is not an every-six-month-checkup kind of deal. You'll be seeing your fertility specialist frequently; in some cases, such as IVF, you may be seeing the specialist almost every day. Look within a reasonable driving radius first.

- ✔ **Convenience:** Fertility treatment often involves frequent blood and ultrasound monitoring. Does the clinic have on-site facilities? (Most do.) Does it have convenient hours? Can you run in for testing and still get to work on time?

- ✔ **Personality:** Fertility clinics, like any type of facility, have their own personalities, starting with the doctors but also including the ancillary personnel such as nurses, lab techs, and front-desk people. Fertility patients often have much of their contact time with nurses. Although it's impossible to evaluate whether you're going to mesh with a clinic until you actually go there, try to get a feel for the place on your first appointment.

✔ **Reputation:** Unless you have an "in" with medical personnel, reputation can be hard to determine. The Centers for Disease Control (CDC) makes it easier to determine a clinic's success rates by publishing assisted reproductive technology statistics for every certified facility in the country every two years; check out www.cdc.gov/art/ARTReports.htm for reports on the clinics you're considering. However, keep in mind that centers that are very picky about who they'll take as patients often have better stats than groups that work with the most difficult patients and have artificially inflated success rates.

Meeting the doctor

Have a list of questions ready before you meet the doctor on your first visit so you won't forget anything. Bring your partner if possible, so he can get his questions answered at the same time. Put the following questions on your list, as well as any others that occur to you:

✔ **What treatments do you suggest starting with?** If your Fallopian tubes are blocked or your partner has major sperm issues, IVF will be your starting point.

✔ **What kind of success rate do you have with people like me?** After all, this is the thing you really want to know before spending thousands of dollars.

✔ **How long should we try one method before moving on to more advanced treatment?** Even if you're starting with IVF, if you don't get pregnant, you can move on to trying donor egg or sperm, or a gestational carrier if circumstances warrant it.

Your doctor will have his own list of questions, although hopefully the doctor knows them well enough not to have to write them down! Be prepared to answer these as well as others:

✔ How long have you been trying to get pregnant?

✔ Have you ever been pregnant? (Don't lie about this one — it's important!)

✔ How often do you have sex?

✔ How often do your periods come?

✔ Are your periods heavy, long, light, or scant?

✔ When was your last period?

✔ Have you had any gynecological problems (such as fibroids, infections, abnormal pap tests, and so on)?

✔ Have you had any abdominal surgery or infections (including appendicitis)?

✔ Does your partner have any health issues or past surgeries (such as hernia repair)? Does he use any drugs or alcohol? Has he ever fathered a child or gotten someone pregnant? (Answer honestly, touchy as it may be.)

✔ Do you have any other health issues?

Going Through Fertility Treatment

Fertility treatment can be long, frustrating, expensive, and ultimately nonproductive if you don't get pregnant. Add to that mix the potent hormones you may be injecting yourself with every day, and fertility treatment can be a minefield for maintaining emotional stability. Knowing what to expect can help you get through the minefield without blowing up on a daily basis.

Testing, testing, testing

Any testing you haven't already had will be done when you get on the fertility treatment merry-go-round. Most centers will accept testing you had done elsewhere, but some will want to repeat certain tests, like the semen analysis, to look for things they deem important that may not have been checked.

Before you start fertility treatment, most centers also require a round of infectious blood work, to make sure you don't have sexually transmitted infections that need treatment before starting fertility procedures. Most also check for HIV and hepatitis B and C. Different centers have different policies on treating women and partners with these disorders.

Learning to inject

Because most fertility medications can't be taken orally, you — or your partner — must learn how to give injections. Most facilities have classes that teach you how to give injections.

The anticipation of learning how to give injections is, in many cases, worse than the actual injection itself. Most fertility medication can be given *subcutaneously* (under the skin), like diabetic medications. The needle is very tiny. You can inject yourself in the top of the leg, or your partner can inject into the fleshy part of the back of your arm.

The only medication that is usually injected intramuscularly, with a longer needle, is human chorionic gonadoptropin (hCG), which is given to ensure that the egg matures and releases from the ovary. Some forms of hCG can be given subcutaneously as well.

Hello, it's me again: Monitoring

Fertility treatment involves frequent monitoring and phone calls to find out your results. Medication doses are often adjusted depending on your response, which is determined by rises in your hormone levels and the growth of follicles seen on ultrasound.

When you're having monitoring done, callback with your results often turns into the most anticipated time of the day. Although most ultrasonographers will share what they see while they're looking at your ovaries, lab techs can't tell anything by looking at your blood, so you need to wait for your callback for the results.

In some centers, doctors make the callbacks, but in many, if not most, nurses do the calls. If you want a callback from your doctor to discuss the results, just ask — but rest assured that the doctor has made the decision on what to do even she isn't actually the one making the phone call.

Types of procedures

Fertility treatments run the gamut from a cycle of Clomid (covered earlier in this chapter) to IVF with donor egg and donor sperm. If you're doing injectable medications because you didn't ovulate with Clomid, you're either doing a medicated cycle (which can be done with or without intrauterine insemination) or an IVF cycle.

Medicated cycles

Injectable medications, called *gonadotropins,* are taken once or twice a day, starting a few days after the first day of your period. Ultrasounds and blood work keep track of how many follicles you're producing and if your hormones are rising appropriately. Each follicle generally contains one egg.

Blood work and ultrasound are necessary for two reasons:

✔ To make sure that you're making follicles

✔ To make sure you're not making too many follicles, a problem that can easily occur in women with PCOS

If your estradiol level rises too high, usually over 1,500 or more in a medicated cycle, you can develop ovarian hyperstimulation syndrome (OHSS), a potentially life-threatening complication in serious cases and one that can make you very ill in any case.

If you start to hyperstimulate, your doctor may cut back on your medications to try to control it. If that doesn't work, he may suggest one of two things:

✔ **Canceling your cycle:** OHSS doesn't develop until after you've ovulated or the eggs have been retrieved. Stopping the cycle can stop OHSS from developing.

✔ **Converting to IVF:** Eggs can be removed from the follicles, fertilized, and frozen for another cycle. Getting pregnant with OHSS increases your chances of developing serious complications. (See the "Recognizing special concerns for women with PCOS" section, later in this chapter, for the risks of OHSS.)

When your follicles look mature, you may get an injection of hCG to ensure that they mature and release properly. If your partner has sperm issues, you may have an IUI, where sperm are washed and concentrated before being placed into the uterus. No, sperm are not inherently dirty — they need washing to remove substances that are normally removed as they transverse the vagina and cervix. If you have no sperm issues, you'll be instructed to have sex at a certain time (no one will follow up to make sure you actually do this) and possibly start taking progesterone to help prepare your uterus for implantation.

Moving up to IVF

IVF is a medicated cycle with the extra twist of an egg retrieval at the end of it. Most fertility doctors don't rush right into IVF unless there's a good reason for it with PCOS patients, although around 15 percent of IVF patients have ovulatory issues. (Pick up a copy of *Infertility For Dummies*, by Sharon Perkins, RN, and Jackie Meyers-Thompson [Wiley], for much more about IVF and other fertility issues.)

Good reasons to move right to IVF include the following:

✔ **Blocked Fallopian tubes:** If your tubes are blocked, the sperm can't reach the egg and the egg can't possibly reach the uterus. The only way you'll get pregnant is with IVF. Previous infection, ectopic pregnancy, or tubal ligation are the most common causes of blocked tubes.

✔ **Very poor sperm quality:** If your partner's sperm count is very low or if the sperm are not motile, doing IVF is the way to go. Sperm and egg are put together in the same dish, so sperm don't have far to go. Another possibility is ICSI, in which one sperm is injected directly into each egg. Although this seems like a surefire way to ensure an embryo, ICSI doesn't always work, because either the egg or the sperm may be chromosomally abnormal.

Looking for success

Although it seems like IVF should be a guarantee of pregnancy (after all, an embryo is created and put right into the uterus where it belongs), it isn't: The embryo may be abnormal. IVF statistics vary according to age; although centers vary considerably and your fertility factors also can have an effect, Table 11-1 lists what you can generally expect.

Table 11-1	Success Rates of IVF based on Age
Age of the Mother	**Success Rate**
34 and under	37%
35 to 37	30%
38 to 40	22%
40 to 42	11%
43 to 44	4%
45 and over	Almost no chance

Understanding what's happening next

The first part of the IVF cycle goes very much like a medicated cycle: You take drugs and get monitored. But after you have a mature follicle (or, more likely, a crop of them), you'll be instructed to take hCG to get your follicles ready for fertilization.

At this point, the procedures take a different path from a medicated cycle. The goal of IVF is to get to the eggs before they ovulate, so the egg retrieval is scheduled for around 34 to 36 hours after you take hCG. The IVF staff will tell you exactly when to do the injection. Follow their instructions. If you take hCG too late, the eggs won't mature before the retrieval and they might not come loose from the ovary. If you take hCG too early, you may ovulate before the retrieval and lose everything.

HCG administration is one of the most crucial parts of the entire retrieval, so do it correctly. If you have any questions on how to mix and administer the hCG, make sure you ask when you get your instructions. Double-check your meds to make sure you have both the hCG and the syringe you need to inject it.

Retrieving the egg

You're not going to hear the staff say when they get eggs during the retrieval, because you will, in nearly all cases, be asleep. Egg retrievals are done by inserting a needle through the back of the vagina into the ovary, so you *want* to be asleep. The anesthesia may be mild IV sedation or Propofol, a stronger drug that must be administered by an anesthesiologist or nurse-anesthetist.

When you're comfortable, fluid is removed from every follicle and given to the embryology staff, who looks for eggs in the fluid. While you're just lying there, your partner is producing his specimen in a separate room.

After the retrieval, you're given some time to wake up and become stable; staff will check your blood pressure and watch for signs of bleeding. After an hour or so, you're free to go. Later in the day, eggs and sperm are mixed together and left overnight, or ICSI is done by the embryology staff. You'll know how many eggs you got right after the retrieval, but you won't know how many embryos you have until the next morning.

Transferring the embryo

Embryos are given a few days to grow in the laboratory before they're transferred back in the uterus. They aren't put back right away because your uterus isn't ready for them yet. It takes a few days for a fertilized egg to reach the uterus in normal fertilization. If the embryo gets there too fast, the uterus isn't prepared for it to implant. Starting progesterone supplements after egg retrieval helps prepare the uterine lining.

Centers do embryo transfers anywhere from two to five days after the egg retrieval. (Different centers have different philosophies on the timing.) The embryos are inserted through a long catheter into the uterus; some centers give valium for the transfer to reduce cramping. Some centers have you lie still for an hour and rest for several days after the transfer; others don't feel it makes any difference. Either way, around ten days after the embryo transfer, you'll get a pregnancy test done and wait for the call from your clinic while biting your nails.

It's probably a rare woman who doesn't do a home pregnancy test — if not a dozen or more — before her blood test. If you test too early, you may get a false positive result from the hCG that stays in your body for ten days or so after you took it. And if your pregnancy levels (known as a beta hCG) are too low for the home pregnancy test to detect, you could still be pregnant. Bottom line: If you do take a test, take the results with a grain of salt. If you're ten days from your transfer and you get a positive result on the home pregnancy test, congratulations! You're definitely pregnant.

Recognizing special concerns for women with PCOS

PCOS can cause special concerns in IVF beyond the risk of hyperstimulation:

- ✔ **Egg quality:** Women with PCOS often have issues with poor egg quality. This is something that you'd know only if you did IVF, where the embryologists get an up-close-and-personal look at your eggs. Poor egg quality often translates into poor fertilization and low pregnancy rates.

  The reasons for poor egg quality in PCOS aren't completely clear, but high insulin levels may be one explanation. Overexposure to the male hormone testosterone also may cause poor egg quality.

  Poor egg quality also contributes to miscarriage. (See Chapter 12 for more on miscarriage and PCOS.)

- ✔ **Hyperstimulation:** Ovarian hyperstimulation syndrome, which causes fluid shifts in the body, occurs in approximately 1 percent to 5 percent of all medicated cycles where gonadotropins are taken. Complications of OHSS include fluid retention, weight gain, headache, weakness, fainting, loss of appetite, difficulty breathing, or abdominal pain. In the most serious cases, blood clots can develop and travel to your lungs, causing a pulmonary embolism.

  Keep your doctor informed of any potential signs of OHSS, especially if you had a large number of eggs retrieved or an estradiol level of over 1,500. Both medicated cycles and IVF cycles may be canceled if your doctor feels the risk of hyperstimulation is too great.

Coping with Disappointment

Months without results, particularly if you're paying dearly for the privilege, can put a huge strain on your relationship with your partner as well as your own mental state. If none of your friends or family has ever gone through infertility, you may not feel like you can talk to them about what you're going through. Even your partner may not "get it," because he can go about his normal life much more easily than you can when you're undergoing infertility treatments.

Fortunately, there's a whole world of women going through the same thing, and you can easily connect with them online in chat rooms and forums. Other websites can keep you informed about your condition and all the newest treatments and research. Check out the following sites to help you keep going on the days when you're feeling like you can't do this alone any longer:

- ✔ **Preconception.com:** Preconception.com is part of iParenting. com which covers all aspects of parenting. Preconception. com offers information for couples trying to conceive.

- ✔ **The Infertility Network (www.ein.org):** The Infertility Network is a nonprofit organization that provides information about infertility and the work of infertility support associations around the world. Its mission is to provide quality up-to-date information and news on assisted reproduction technology, infertility, getting pregnant, and other aspects of infertility.

- ✔ **American Society for Reproductive Medicine (ASRM; www. asrm.org):** ASRM is interested in all aspects of the reproductive lifecycle. It provides information on infertility, menopause, contraception, reproductive surgery, endometriosis, and other reproductive issues. ASRM can provide you with fact sheets and questions on topics related to reproductive health.

- ✔ **International Council of Infertility Information Dissemination (INCID; www.inciid.org):** INCIID (pronounced "inside") is a nonprofit organization that helps individuals and couples explore their family-building options. INCIID provides current information and immediate support regarding the diagnosis, treatment, and prevention of infertility and pregnancy loss, and offers guidance to those considering adoption or child-free lifestyles.

- ✔ **RESOLVE (www.resolve.org):** The mission of RESOLVE is to provide support and information to people who are experiencing infertility and to increase awareness of infertility issues through public education and advocacy.

- ✔ **Fertility Research Foundation (FRF; www.frfbaby.com):** Established in 1964, FRF provides fertility counseling and treatments.

Chapter 12

Pregnancy Complications and PCOS

• •

In This Chapter

▶ Deciding if you need a doctor who specializes in high-risk pregnancies

▶ Paying attention to the foods you eat

▶ Identifying complicating factors when you have PCOS

▶ Dealing with diabetes in pregnancy

▶ Watching your blood pressure

▶ Handling the risks of preterm delivery

• •

*I*f you have PCOS, it may have taken a lot of blood, sweat, and tears to get to the point where you are now — looking at that little stick with a big plus sign in the middle or taking the call from your fertility clinic with the news that your blood test was positive.

Although we'd love to say that you can sit back, relax, and enjoy the next nine months without giving PCOS a thought, that's not the case — PCOS can affect many aspects of your pregnancy. The more you know what to look for and how to prevent complications, the easier your pregnancy will hopefully be. This chapter helps you prepare.

Choosing a Doctor

If you have PCOS, choosing a doctor to see you through pregnancy may take a bit more thought than usual. You may or may not be considered a "high-risk" obstetric patient, depending on the complications of PCOS you already have.

Doctors who specialize in high-risk obstetrics are called *perinatologists*. You may want to consider seeing a perinatologist if:

✔ You have diabetes.

✔ You're having *multiples* (more than one baby), common after infertility treatment.

✔ You have high blood pressure.

✔ You have any type of heart disease.

A perinatologist may or may not attend your delivery. In some cases, the perinatologist follows you during pregnancy and works with your obstetrician to prevent complications but does not actually do deliveries. In other cases, the perinatologist may also be the doctor who attends your delivery.

Eating Well to Prevent Pregnancy Complications

Getting the nutrients you need during pregnancy is important. Even though overweight women have more pregnancy complications than women of normal weight, pregnancy or the time when you're trying to get pregnant is not the time to diet. Women who conceive while dieting are more likely to have low-birth-weight babies. These babies are much more likely to have immediate as well as long-term health problems (see the nearby sidebar "Low-birth-weight babies are at risk").

When it comes to vitamin and mineral supplements, in some cases, more is not better. A prenatal vitamin with iron is usually enough for most pregnant women, but follow your doctor's recommendation.

Getting extra folic acid

Congenital diseases such as *spina bifida* (an abnormal opening in the spine) and *anencephaly* (the absence of a large part of the brain and skull) are called *neural tube defects*. Neural tube defects can be the result of having too little folate (one of the B vitamins) in the diet. The neural tube is formed well before a woman realizes she's pregnant. Neural tube defects occur when the brain and skull and/or the spinal cord and its protective spinal column don't develop properly within the first few weeks after conception, so having enough of this vitamin is critical before conception and during the first 12 weeks of pregnancy.

Low-birth-weight babies are at risk

In addition to causing problems with fertility, not adopting a healthy lifestyle before you conceive puts you at risk of having a low-birth-weight baby. *Low birth weight* is defined as under 5½ pounds. A low-birth-weight infant is at risk for the following:

- Congenital malformations, particularly of the central nervous system
- Low intelligence
- Behavioral problems
- Reduced immunity
- Increased risk of developing allergies

Some experts believe that low birth weight also may predispose your baby to diseases such as high blood pressure and diabetes.

To safeguard the baby, women who are planning a pregnancy should take a daily 400-microgram supplement of *folic acid* (the manufactured form of folate, which is easily absorbed by the body and acts in the same way as folate does in food). In addition, women should also consume plenty of folate-rich foods (such as most beans or lentils; vegetables such as broccoli, beets, Brussels sprouts, and spinach; and fruit such as tomatoes and avocados). Foods fortified with folic acid, such as breakfast cereals and other grain products, also help boost folic acid intake.

Avoiding extra vitamins

Although having enough of the essential vitamins and minerals in the diet is important, taking excessive amounts of some of these can be harmful to you and to a potential baby.

One such vitamin is vitamin A. Vitamin A in the diet is derived from two sources:

- As vitamin A precursors called *carotenoids*, which are found in many fruits and vegetables
- As retinol, which is a preformed form of vitamin A and is found in some animal products such as dairy products, liver, and fish liver oil

Animal livers contain very high levels of retinol. (This is thought to be because retinol is added to the animal feed to enhance productivity, reproduction, and immune status.) Therefore, experts advise women who are pregnant or may become pregnant to avoid the following:

- ✔ Liver and liver products (such as pâtés)
- ✔ Supplements containing retinol (including high-dose multivitamins)
- ✔ Cod-liver oil supplements

Only the preformed variety of vitamin A is dangerous. High amounts are toxic to the developing baby and can cause birth defects. The same is true if you take high-dose supplements of retinol, so experts have set a limit of 3,000 micrograms per day.

A recent study published in the respected medical journal *The Lancet* showed that high doses of vitamins C and E taken during pregnancy actually increase the risk of having a baby with a low birth weight. However, researchers confirmed that doses of these antioxidant vitamins taken in the amounts found in multivitamin supplements didn't pose a threat.

Protecting yourself from food poisoning

Food poisoning is an unpleasant experience for anyone, but if you're pregnant, some food-borne diseases can harm the baby before you're even aware that you're pregnant. Furthermore, a food-borne disease can lurk in the body for a long while. It can take up to three months to establish adequate immunity from these diseases, which means that your newly conceived baby is left unprotected.

Here are some general rules on food hygiene that are good to follow in general but especially if you're planning to get pregnant:

- ✔ Store food as directed by the food manufacturer.
- ✔ Eat food by the "use by" date.
- ✔ Store raw food on the bottom shelf of the fridge so that juices from the raw food don't drip on anything else.
- ✔ Use separate chopping boards for raw and cooked foods.
- ✔ Cook all food thoroughly and avoid eating shellfish or raw or undercooked fish, meat, eggs, or poultry.
- ✔ When reheating food, make sure that it's piping hot all the way through. Don't reheat food more than once.

✔ Cooked food that is not eaten right away should be cooled as rapidly as possible and then stored in the refrigerator.

✔ Avoid unpasteurized milk and milk products.

✔ Avoid foods that carry a high risk of being contaminated with listeria. Listeria can cause *listeriosis,* a disease that can lead to miscarriage, stillbirth, or sickness in a newborn infant. Listeria also can make a pregnant woman extremely ill or even lead to death.

Foods that can cause listeria include the following:

- Soft, ripened cheese such as brie, Camembert, or blue-vein cheeses.

- Processed meats such as cold cuts. Thoroughly cook all prepackaged meats, which may become contaminated during processing after cooking but before packaging.

- Prepackaged supermarket salads.

- Salads in dressings from deli counters.

Early Pregnancy Complications and PCOS

Women with PCOS may develop several complications in early pregnancy. Some potential complications, such as multiple births, occur more frequently in women who undergo fertility treatment. Others, like a higher risk of early miscarriage, are problems that affect women with PCOS in general.

Multiple birth and fertility treatments

Assisted reproductive technologies such as in vitro fertilization (IVF) and intrauterine insemination or fertility medications such as Clomid or injectable gonadotropins can all increase your risk of having more than one baby. (See Chapter 11 for more about the various fertility treatments available that may be helpful if you have PCOS.)

If you're hoping to have more than one child eventually, the possibility of twins may actually seem like a bonus, especially if you're paying for expensive fertility treatments out-of-pocket. But two for the price of one can increase you risk of complications in pregnancy, and three — or more — for the price of one can have significant risks for the babies as well.

The natural twinning rate is around 1 in 80 pregnancies. Among Clomid users, between 6 percent and 10 percent end up with multiple pregnancies. For women who undergo IVF procedures, around 31 percent deliver multiples, with 24 percent having twins, 8 percent triplets, and less than 1 percent quads or more. Around 17 percent of all twins and 40 percent of triplets are the result of fertility treatments of some type.

Some of the increased risks of multiple pregnancy include the following:

- **Preterm delivery:** As many as 60 percent of twin pregnancies deliver before 37 weeks, and 12 percent deliver before 32 weeks. Around 36 percent of triplets deliver before 32 weeks. Around 80 percent of quads or higher-order multiples deliver before 32 weeks.

- **Low birth weight:** More than 50 percent of all babies born from multiple pregnancies weigh less than 5½ pounds.

- **Increased risk of complications such as pregnancy-induced hypertension, pre-eclampsia, or gestational diabetes.**

Not all multiple pregnancies will continue; in fact, as many as 21 percent to 30 percent of pregnancies that start out as multiples end up as singletons, a syndrome known as *vanishing twin syndrome*. For women who aren't undergoing fertility treatments, this often happens before they even realize they're pregnant. But when you're undergoing fertility treatment, you normally find out you're pregnant very early on, so you're more likely to be aware if you were pregnant with multiples and lost one. This experience can be devastating and result in a sense of loss even when you're still pregnant with one baby.

Miscarriage

Women with PCOS have a higher risk of miscarriage than those without PCOS. The reasons for this have not been thoroughly established. As many 30 percent to 50 percent of women who conceive with PCOS miscarry, according to some studies.

Although this sounds extremely high, it's important to remember that as many as 25 percent of all pregnancies end in miscarriage, regardless of whether a woman has PCOS. Many of these losses occur before the woman even realizes that she's pregnant. Because women with PCOS often undergo fertility treatment, they may have pregnancy testing done much earlier than most women would.

Determining the causes

Some of the possible causes for the increased rate of miscarriage in women with PCOS are a number of hormonal imbalances, including the following:

- ✔ **High levels of male hormones such as testosterone:** Women with high testosterone levels appear to have a higher miscarriage rate than those with normal levels.

- ✔ **Higher prolactin levels:** Women with PCOS may have higher-than-normal prolactin levels during the early part of the menstrual cycle, called the *follicular phase*.

- ✔ **High levels of luteinizing hormone (LH):** Women with PCOS often have a higher-than-normal LH-to-FSH (follicle stimulating hormone) ratio. Because LH is responsible for the egg releasing from the follicle, high LH levels may cause arrested development in the egg, which may, in turn, cause chromosomal abnormalities.

- ✔ **Luteal phase defect:** If the developing follicle isn't stimulated by high enough FSH levels during the follicular phase, the *corpus luteum* (the leftover "shell" of the follicle that remains after ovulation) may not develop properly. The corpus luteum produces progesterone, which prepares the uterine lining for implantation. If the corpus luteum doesn't develop, progesterone levels may be too low to support a growing embryo.

Insulin resistance also can contribute to a higher-than-normal miscarriage rate in women with PCOS. Insulin stimulates release of LH and testosterone, and high levels of both can increase the risk of miscarriage.

Recognizing the symptoms

If miscarriage occurs very early in pregnancy, before you've even missed a period, the only sign may be a heavier-than-normal menstrual period that may come a few days late — or right on time. Many early miscarriages are never recognized, even in women who don't have PCOS.

If you've already had a positive pregnancy test, the following signs may occur before a miscarriage:

- ✔ A lessening of pregnancy symptoms, such as sore breasts or nausea.

- ✔ *Spotting* (passage of small amounts of brownish mucus or bright red blood).

✔ Cramping, usually more than the cramping of a regular menstrual period. Cramping intensifies if your cervix starts to open and the embryo is expelled.

Diagnosing a miscarriage

If you have symptoms of miscarriage, your doctor may suggest doing a pelvic ultrasound. If you're between six and seven weeks pregnant, a fetal heartbeat can usually be seen on ultrasound. If a heartbeat is seen at or after seven weeks and the hormone levels are normal, the risk of miscarriage is very low. Other causes of bleeding, such as a *sub-chorionic hematoma* (a blood clot in the placenta), may be visible on ultrasound.

Your levels of human chorionic gonadotropin (hCG), the hormone produced by the placenta during pregnancy, may rise more slowly or begin to fall if the pregnancy is not viable. (You would only know this if you've been having bloodwork done every few days.)

If a heartbeat was previously seen and is no longer visible, but you haven't started bleeding and your cervix isn't open, your doctor may say you've have had a missed abortion. Despite the unfortunate choice of terminology, an *abortion* in medical terms simply means a pregnancy loss. A missed abortion may require a surgical procedure called a *dilatation and curettage* (D&C) to remove the products of conception. If this isn't done, you could develop an infection.

Treating a miscarriage

In most cases, it's not possible to prevent miscarriage from occurring. Statistically, most miscarriages are caused by chromosomally abnormal embryos. The roots of many hormone imbalances are in the first part of the menstrual cycle, even before ovulation occurs. The hormonal imbalances that can lead to miscarriage generally can't be corrected after symptoms of miscarriage appear.

Doctors usually don't recommend bed rest for a threatened miscarriage. Because normal physical activity is not the cause of the bleeding or other symptoms, bed rest won't stop a miscarriage from happening.

Trying again

Doctors don't normally consider miscarriage as a sign you'll have difficulty carrying a baby to term unless you've had three or more miscarriages. Most doctors suggest waiting until one month after you've had a normal period after a miscarriage before trying again. The risk of miscarriage if you get pregnant without having a regular period between pregnancies can increase the miscarriage rate by one and a half times.

Hands off the litter box

Toxoplasmosis is a particularly nasty parasite that can be carried by household pets, especially cats. If you become infected with this parasite in the very early stages of pregnancy or just before you get pregnant, toxoplasmosis can lead to blindness and other problems in your baby.

You can take some simple actions to avoid picking up this parasite:

✓ Avoid changing cat litter, or wear rubber gloves and disinfect them afterward.

✓ Wear gloves when gardening because the parasite can live in soil where the cat has defecated.

✓ Wash your hands after handling pets.

Expect to have bleeding for several weeks after a miscarriage, although it should slow to spotting within a few days. If bleeding becomes heavy or if you have foul-smelling vaginal discharge, call your doctor.

Preventing another miscarriage

Medications to decrease insulin resistance may help prevent a miscarriage related to out-of-whack hormones by reducing levels of LH, testosterone, and insulin. Ask your doctor about taking metformin while trying to get pregnant and during pregnancy. At least one study has shown that continuing metformin throughout pregnancy reduced miscarriage rates from 36 percent to 11 percent, in addition to reducing the chances of developing gestational diabetes. In one small study, only 3 percent of women with PCOS developed gestational diabetes when taking metformin compared to 23 percent of those not taking metformin. (See Chapter 11 for more about metformin.)

Dealing with Diabetes

Because women with PCOS have an increased risk of diabetes in general, it should come as no surprise that pregnant women with PCOS have a higher risk of developing gestational diabetes. In addition, some women with PCOS already may have type 2 diabetes before they get pregnant. Diabetes can have a major impact on your pregnancy and on your baby.

Diabetes before pregnancy

If you already have diabetes, it's important to remember that your baby's major organs all form during the first eight weeks of pregnancy. High levels of glucose during early pregnancy can cause birth defects. Damage done during this early stage can't be reversed, so make sure your blood glucose levels are under good control before getting pregnant.

Gestational diabetes also can increase the risk of birth defects, but only if you have a body mass index (BMI) over 25 at the start of pregnancy. (See Chapter 4 for more about BMI.) Birth defects caused by uncontrolled blood sugar levels can be severe and include the following:

- Brain and spinal defects such as spina bifida
- Cleft lip or palate
- Heart defects
- Kidney or gastrointestinal-tract defects
- Limb deficiencies

Keep the statistics in perspective, though. Having diabetes doesn't mean your child will have birth defects. In one study, having type 1 or type 2 diabetes before pregnancy doubled the risk of having a child with birth defects. But birth defects can occur from many causes. In one study, around 93 percent of all children born with birth defects were born to mothers who did *not* have diabetes before pregnancy.

Developing gestational diabetes

As many as 4 percent to 10 percent of women develop gestational diabetes, but the percentage is higher in women with PCOS. Having PCOS may increase your risk of developing gestational diabetes more than threefold, according to some studies. Other experts put the risk at 40 percent for women with PCOS. Being overweight at the start of pregnancy is also a risk factor for developing gestational diabetes.

Gestational diabetes is generally diagnosed by a glucose screening test, sometimes called a glucose challenge test, between 24 and 28 weeks of pregnancy, but testing may be done sooner if you have risk factors such as:

- Being obese at the start of pregnancy, with a BMI over 30.
- Having an elevated fasting blood glucose level of over 100 mg/dL.

✔ Spilling sugar into your urine. (This is one of the things that your doctor checks your urine for at every visit.)

A glucose screening test is done as follows:

1. **You drink or eat a 50-gram glucose solution after having a fasting blood sugar drawn.**

2. **An hour later, your blood is drawn again.**

   A level between 130 mg/dL or 140 mg/dL (depending on the lab) and 200 mg/dL is considered a gray area, and you'll need to take a three-hour glucose tolerance test.

3. **If your glucose level is over 200 mg/dL, you'll be diagnosed with gestational diabetes without undergoing further testing.**

A three-hour glucose tolerance test (GTT) is similar to the glucose challenge test, but blood is drawn at one-, two-, and three-hour intervals. The following levels are considered abnormal:

✔ **At one hour:** 180 mg/dL or higher

✔ **At two hours:** 155 mg/dL or higher

✔ **At three hours:** 140 mg/dL or higher

Complications for the baby

Infants whose mothers have either diabetes or gestational diabetes are at increased risk for complications during and after delivery. The main risk for infants of diabetic mothers is *macrosomia* (larger-than-normal size). Although being bigger than normal at birth doesn't seem like such a bad thing (many parents actually brag about how big their babies were), big babies have a harder time making it through the birth canal and also have a harder time maintaining their blood sugars after delivery because they've become used to a steady stream of sugar-rich nutrients delivered through the placenta. There is also an increased risk of birth defects.

Newborns who are used to a higher level of blood glucose than other babies can become jittery and develop tremors or other signs of low blood sugar, called *hypoglycemia,* after delivery. They often need to be watched closely to make sure they don't develop signs of hypoglycemia, which in severe cases can lead to brain damage in newborns.

Newborns are also more likely to have jaundice and respiratory distress syndrome (RDS), which makes it harder for them to breathe normally. They also can have low calcium and magnesium levels. Babies born with low calcium or magnesium levels may be jittery and develop seizures.

Keeping blood glucose levels under control during pregnancy is a major part of avoiding macrosomia. Work with a dietitian or your medical provider to devise a diet plan that provides good nutrition while keeping your blood sugars as close to normal as possible. You may have to take metformin or insulin injections during the pregnancy to achieve this.

Delivery complications

The most dreaded complication for large babies at the time of delivery is *shoulder dystocia*. Babies with shoulder dystocia have shoulders that are wider than their head circumference. Normally, a baby's head is his widest part, so if his head makes it through the birth canal, the rest of the baby does, too. But babies with shoulder dystocia get their heads out and then get their shoulders hung up on the pubic bone.

Shoulder dystocia is one of the most dangerous and frightening complications of delivery. To get the baby out of the birth canal can require maneuvers that can fracture the baby's collarbone or damage the nerves in the arm, resulting in an injury called *brachial plexus palsy*. A baby who gets stuck in the birth canal also may become oxygen deprived because the umbilical cord is compressed. If your obstetrician is concerned that your baby may be too big to navigate the birth canal, she may plan to do a Cesarean section to deliver your baby.

Overall, babies born to diabetic mothers have the following delivery risks:

✔ Twice the risk of serious birth injury

✔ Three times the rate of Cesarean section

✔ Four times the risk of admission to neonatal intensive care

Handling High Blood Pressure

High blood pressure, like high blood sugar, can cause serious complications in pregnancy, including pregnancy loss and maternal death, in rare cases. Women who are overweight and who have high blood pressure before pregnancy are most likely to develop serious blood pressure complications during pregnancy. Make sure to follow your medical provider's recommendations for keeping blood pressure under control during pregnancy. You may need to limit salt intake as well as take medications to control your blood pressure.

Gestational hypertension

Most studies show that women with PCOS have an increased risk of developing gestational hypertension (GH, previously known as pregnancy-induced hypertension, or PIH), but some studies have not established a definite increased risk. Studies peg the risk anywhere from three times the normal risk to a 12 percent risk for women with PCOS (compared to a 1.3 percent risk for women without PCOS). Being overweight, being insulin resistant, and having borderline blood pressure before pregnancy all increase the risk, even in women without PCOS.

Gestational hypertension is high blood pressure that develops after the 20th week of pregnancy. The most severe forms of GH are known as pre-eclampsia or toxemia of pregnancy. GH is characterized by the following:

- ✔ **Blood pressure greater than 140/90** or readings that are higher than pre-pregnancy readings

- ✔ **Protein in the urine**

- ✔ *Edema* **(fluid retention that causes swelling),** especially in the extremities, hands, and feet.

Severe GH can cause sudden weight gain, headaches, nausea or vomiting, upper-right-quadrant abdominal pain, decreased urination, abnormal liver enzymes, blurred vision, light sensitivity, or hyperactive reflexes.

If not treated, GH can lead to a number of complications, including:

- ✔ *Eclampsia* **(the development of seizures, possible coma, and fetal or maternal death in severe cases):** Delivery of the baby is the only cure for severe GH, although magnesium sulfate infusions may help reduce the risk of seizures and lower blood pressure in some cases.

- ✔ **Placental abruption:** High blood pressure can cause the placenta to prematurely detach from the uterine wall, cutting off the baby's oxygen supply and causing maternal hemorrhage.

- ✔ **Intrauterine growth retardation:** High blood pressure can decrease blood flow through the placenta, which decreases nutrient delivery to the fetus. The baby may not grow well.

✔ **Stillbirth:** Decreased blood flow through the placenta could lead to fetal death.

✔ **HELLP syndrome:** HELLP stands for *hemolysis–elevated liver enzymes–low platelets,* all of which describe the symptoms of this rare but potentially deadly complication of severe GH.

Preterm Delivery

The various complications of PCOS in pregnancy can lead to *preterm delivery,* defined as delivery before 37 weeks of pregnancy. Although just about every pregnant woman is sick of being pregnant during the last few weeks and eager to deliver, premature delivery can have a number of harmful effects on a newborn, including the following:

✔ **Respiratory problems:** Because their lungs aren't fully developed, premature babies often have breathing problems. The more premature a baby is, the more severe the problems may be and the longer she'll need treatments such as oxygen supplementation or artificial ventilation.

✔ **Feeding problems:** Tiny babies, under 28 weeks, may not be fed by mouth for weeks or even months, because their digestive system isn't well enough developed to digest food. Intravenous feedings will be given instead, and as the baby grows, feeding through a tube that goes directly to the baby's stomach through the mouth or nose may be started. Bottle- or breast-feeding takes additional energy and can burn too many calories in preemies, even if they can suck and swallow at the same time, a reflex that doesn't develop until around the 30th week of pregnancy.

✔ **Infections:** Preemies don't have well-developed immune systems and may not be able to fight off infections well.

Keeping Things in Perspective

Looking at all the things that can go wrong during pregnancy when you have PCOS can be so frightening, you may decide to forget the whole idea. But take heart: If you keep blood glucose levels under control, eat well, and lose even a small amount of weight before getting pregnant, you can significantly decrease your risk of complications during pregnancy.

Most women with PCOS go through pregnancy without any complications at all, and you can increase your chances of being one of them by getting into the best shape possible before trying to get pregnant.

Part IV
The Part of Tens

The 5th Wave   By Rich Tennant

"Oh, I have a very healthy relationship with food. It's the relationship I have with my scales that's not so good."

In this part...

The Part of Tens takes one last look at the positive steps you can take to live a happy and productive life even if you have PCOS. In this part, we review the actions you can take to combat symptoms, toss in a few more diet tips and tricks, and show you where you can find more information on PCOS.

Chapter 13

Ten PCOS Symptoms You Can Take Action On

. . . .

In This Chapter

▶ Scoping out the PCOS symptoms you can do something about

▶ Getting motivated to take action to reduce those symptoms

. . . .

Taking control of your diet and lifestyle really helps you to lessen some of the unpleasant side effects of PCOS, in addition to reducing your risk of getting even more serious medical conditions, such as diabetes and heart disease. This chapter lists ten PCOS-related symptoms that you can ameliorate just by being proactive with your health.

Frumpiness and Feeling out of Shape

The answer to feeling frumpy and unfit is easy on paper: You need to tighten up on your diet and do some exercise. Of course, real life is more difficult than that. However, even if you start off just by getting more physically active, you can go a long way toward feeling more toned and fit.

Although exercise alone won't lead to the kind of weight loss you can achieve with the combination of diet and exercise, it *can* make weight loss easier, help you maintain your weight, and offset further weight gain. Exercise can offset feelings of frumpiness by

✔ **Making you feel more energetic for the rest of the day:** Feeling frumpy is harder when you feel energized!

✔ **Lifting your mood and giving you a more positive outlook on life:** When you have a more positive outlook, you aren't as likely to feel down on yourself.

✔ **Toning your whole body:** So, even if you're the same weight, you look slimmer and clothes hang on you better.

✔ **Improving your fitness:** You notice this when you don't get so out of breath walking up the stairs or walking briskly through the mall.

✔ **Helping to reduce your tummy:** The tummy is a real problem area if you have PCOS.

You also need to address frumpiness with diet. The diet you follow should be around 1,500 calories per day. Sticking to low-GI eating (where you eat mostly carbs that have a low glycemic index; see Chapter 4) is also recommended, unless you've been advised differently by a healthcare professional. Don't follow a diet or exercise regime that hasn't been approved by a qualified nurse, dietitian, or doctor.

A steady weight loss of 1 to 2 pounds per week is fine. It may seem frustrating to be losing weight slowly, but you'll get there in the end. The combination of a balanced diet that isn't too strict, coupled with exercise, helps to ensure that you don't lose muscle mass and that the weight stays off.

Trouble Getting Pregnant

PCOS is often diagnosed when you've been trying to get pregnant but haven't been able to. (See Chapters 10 and 11 for more on getting pregnant with PCOS.) In order to restore fertility, you need to stop the whole insulin-resistance cascade from happening at the very start. This means losing weight, which then reduces the overproduction of insulin and reduces hormone imbalances.

The good news is that losing even 5 percent of your current weight (if you're overweight) can trigger a return to fertility. The final effect is that the ovaries release an egg that can be fertilized. And, hopefully, the patter of tiny feet won't be far behind.

Diabetes

Gaining weight, particularly around the middle (which is what tends to happen in PCOS), triggers the production of a hormone that can trigger the muscle cells to be insensitive to the effects of insulin. (See Chapter 3 for more on the effects of insulin in PCOS.) This triggers the pancreas to push out more insulin. Eventually, the cells that produce the insulin get exhausted and can't keep up with the amount of insulin needed to bring blood glucose levels down to a normal level.

When blood glucose levels start to exceed the normal range, this is the point where type 2 diabetes develops. A person with type 2 diabetes whose blood sugars aren't controlled adequately has an increased risk of developing several complications, such as

- ✔ Heart disease and stroke, which are mainly caused by damage to the arteries

- ✔ Kidney damage, which leads to kidney failure

- ✔ Damage to the *retina* (the back of the eye), which can lead to blindness

- ✔ Nerve damage

- ✔ Increased risk of developing gangrene in the feet, which may result in needing to have a foot amputated

To prevent type 2 diabetes from developing, and to lessen its impact if it has already occurred, you have to lose weight and exercise. Even a small weight loss of 5 percent can have a significant effect. If you have type 2 diabetes or insulin resistance, following a low-GI diet helps you to

- ✔ Have better blood sugar control in the short and long term

- ✔ Reduce the diabetic medication needed to control your blood sugar

- ✔ Lose more weight

- ✔ Reduce the risk of developing heart disease and other complications of diabetes

Cancer

The relationship between PCOS and cancer, in general, is not completely clear, although women who are overweight are more likely to get some kinds of cancer. Also, in general, women who are infertile (whether they have PCOS or not) are more likely than fertile women to get a cancer of the reproductive system.

The cancer with the strongest link to PCOS is endometrial cancer, which affects the lining of the uterus. PCOS causes disruptions to the normal menstrual cycle: irregular menstrual periods and the absence of ovulation. Absence of ovulation leads to the production of estrogen, but not progesterone. Without progesterone, the uterine lining doesn't shed but continues to grow. This precancerous condition is called *endometrial hyperplasia,* and if it's allowed to continue over a long period of time, it can develop into full-blown endometrial cancer. (See Chapter 10 for ways to avoid developing endometrial hyperplasia.)

A few studies have suggested a correlation between PCOS and breast cancer; others have not. No relationship seems to exist between PCOS and ovarian cancer. Breast cancer and endometrial cancer are described as "estrogen-sensitive" cancers, meaning that the presence of estrogen may cause these cancer cells to multiply.

So, having a regular period is very important for more than just fertility reasons. Again, the answer here is to lose weight. Even a relatively small weight loss can help to make your periods more regular.

Heart Disease and Stroke

Researchers have found that PCOS — with its symptoms of high blood pressure, excessive fat around the abdominal area, blood fat disorders (such as high triglycerides and low HDL), elevated levels of male hormones, and insulin resistance — puts sufferers at higher risk of developing future serious, life-threatening health conditions such as coronary heart disease and stroke.

Recommendations for reducing your risk of cardiovascular disease involve the following:

✔ Reducing insulin resistance

✔ Reducing the level of "bad" cholesterol (LDL) and raising the level of "good" cholesterol (HDL)

✔ Lowering blood pressure

You need to control your PCOS symptoms as much as possible in order to delay or prevent worsening of the underlying conditions that lead to heart disease. You can do this by being careful in your food choices (lowering caloric intake if you need to lose weight, minimizing your consumption of saturated fat and salt, and following a low-GI diet), and getting regular exercise.

Following a diet that includes plenty of low-GI foods may have a role in helping to prevent or reduce the risk of getting type 2 diabetes. Because diabetes increases your risk of getting heart disease big time, controlling your diet is obviously an important action that you can take yourself. Research also has shown that lower-GI diets can help improve levels of "good" cholesterol and so may reduce the risk of heart disease in general.

Depression

If you have PCOS, you're likely to feel low, depressed, and irritable sometimes. Symptoms of PCOS are similar to that of PMS and have the same root cause: hormonal fluctuations. Low self-esteem from appearance issues, feeling tired, and being overwhelmed by your condition can add to depression. Not getting pregnant when you're trying is also a source of depression. Finally, some medications used to treat PCOS can trigger irritability and depression; ask your doctor if there are alternative drugs that don't increase depression.

If you're not sure whether what you're feeling is true depression, check it out against some of the characteristics of depression:

- ✔ Feeling down for more than a couple days in a row
- ✔ Avoiding having a social life and preferring to stay at home by yourself
- ✔ Crying without obvious provocation
- ✔ Persistent trouble sleeping
- ✔ Being overly critical of yourself
- ✔ Thinking about suicide, and feeling that the world and your family would be better off without you

If you think you're suffering from depression, which is more than feeling down from time to time, see your doctor to get help. You're unlikely to be able to deal with your PCOS in an appropriate way if you're truly depressed. Of course, getting regular exercise and eating a varied, balanced diet will be a big factor in helping you shake it off, but you may also need to take some medication in the short term and receive appropriate therapy.

Unwanted Hair

There aren't too many things that make a woman feel less like a woman than hair growing in places it shouldn't. Sprouting whiskers, feeling like you need a daily shave, or plucking at hair growing on your chest, back, or toes can be both demoralizing and socially embarrassing.

Fortunately, electrolysis, depilatory creams, and waxing can help remove stubborn hairs. In addition, you can reduce the amount of male hormones you have circulating (and, thus, decrease hair growth) by losing weight and taking medications such as birth control pills.

Hair Loss

About 15 percent of women have hair loss, but a significant percentage of those are women with PCOS. As with unwanted hair (see the preceding section), an excess of male hormones is the cause.

Normally, roughly 100 hairs are lost from a person's head every day. The average scalp contains about 100,000 hairs. Hair grows from its follicle at an average rate of about 1/2 inch per month. Each hair grows for two to six years, rests, and then falls out. A new hair soon begins growing in its place. At any one time, about 85 percent of the hair is growing and 15 percent is resting. Hair loss or baldness occurs when hair falls out but new hair doesn't grow in its place.

Loss of hair is more than a minor cosmetic problem. It has the potential to make you feel vulnerable and embarrassed. Women experience hair loss differently than men do. In women, the main patterns are

- ✔ Thinning of hair over the entire head
- ✔ Mild to moderate hair loss at the crown or hairline

Unfortunately, the hair loss of female-pattern baldness or severe thinning may be permanent. So, prevention is essential by restoring normal hormonal levels and reducing insulin resistance.

Messed-Up Periods

The name *polycystic ovary syndrome* comes from the appearance of the ovaries in some women with the disorder: large and studded with numerous cysts. These cysts are fluid-filled sacs, known as *follicles,* which contain immature eggs. Because the eggs never reach maturity, periods get disrupted or stop altogether. Irregular periods, or none at all, are the most common symptom of PCOS.

Four out of five women with PCOS have some sort of period disruption. In PCOS the periods can be

✔ Absent altogether (known medically as *amenorrhea*).

✔ Irregular (known medically as *oligomenorrhea*). Irregular menstruation means having menstrual cycles that occur at intervals longer than 35 days or fewer than eight times a year.

✔ Heavy (known medically as *menorrhagia*).

✔ Last a long time (seven days or more).

Sometimes spotting is present between periods, where the endometrium that has built up does break down to a certain extent, even though no ovulation has occurred.

Fertility is affected if the menstrual cycle is disrupted, because this irregular cycle is an indication that a mature egg is not being released on a monthly basis. If no period occurs, no egg is being released, so conception isn't possible.

One answer to irregular periods is, once again, weight loss, because losing weight enables the hormone levels that disrupt menstruation to return to normal. Keep in mind that this process works in the opposite direction, too: The more weight you gain, the more irregular your periods become, and the more likely you are to stop having periods altogether.

Lack of Energy

You're not imagining it: PCOS really can tire you out. Between the mood swings related to hormone changes, the constant hunger, the lack of energy getting into your cells, and the worry about what's happening to you, days where you don't feel like you have the energy to get out of bed may become the rule rather than the exception.

Life doesn't have to be all worry and no fun, though, even when you have a chronic disease. One way to get a grip on PCOS is to learn all you can about it. This may sound counterintuitive: How can you forget about something when you're learning all you can about it? But the goal isn't to forget you have PCOS — it's to feel like you have a handle on it and that you know what to expect. Worrying about what's going to happen next will have you constantly on edge.

Keep up with all the latest information, do everything you can to improve your symptoms, and you'll feel like you're in control of PCOS, not the other way around.

Chapter 14

Ten Signs to Avoid a Diet

In This Chapter

▶ Knowing when not to touch a diet with a ten-foot pole

▶ Explaining why some diets may be downright dangerous

*Y*ou've probably read, or even tried to follow, many different diets over your lifetime — most women have! Diets are everywhere — friends, relatives, celebrities, books, magazines, newspapers, the Internet. . . . Many of these diets seem attractive because they're a little different from the usual boring diet advice and they claim fantastic results, but that's precisely what makes them dangerous. This chapter gives you signs of diets to avoid.

It Excludes Certain Foods

The key to a good diet is to eat a variety of different foods. That way, you can more or less guarantee that you get all the nutrients your body needs. No one food that you eat is going to be the perfect food, containing the whole assortment of nutrients you need (unless of course it's a specially made-up formula food), which is why you need a whole mixture of foods in your diet.

Diets that restrict you from eating certain foods may cut out foods that provide you with important nutrients. These diets are often hyped up and claim unrealistic results. They normally work by cutting out major food groups (such as carbs in the Atkins diet).

Table 14-1 lists the nutrients you may get too little of if you cut a particular food group out of your diet.

Table 14-1	Food Groups and What They Provide	
Food Group	*Examples of Food Group*	*What the Food Group Provides to the Diet*
Fats	Butter, margarine, oil, fatty meat, cheese	Fat-soluble vitamins and essential fatty acids; also allows absorption of several antioxidants, such as lycopene from tomatoes
Carbohydrates	Pasta, rice, bread, potatoes (ordinary and sweet)	Energy, fiber, B vitamins, magnesium
Dairy	Milk, cheese, yogurt	Calcium; riboflavin (vitamin B2); fat-soluble vitamins such as A, D, and E
Fruits and vegetables	All fruits and vegetables (but not potatoes)	Fiber, antioxidants, vitamins A and C, magnesium
Meat, fish, and other protein sources	Beef, pork, lamb, chicken, white and oily fish, beans, nuts, legumes	Protein, iron, zinc, other minerals

Unless you've been told to exclude certain foods for medical reasons (such as avoiding eggs or nuts due to an allergy), don't omit any particular food from your diet. If you choose to avoid a particular food, make sure that you replace it with something that provides the same nutrients. For example, if you cut meat out of your diet, you need to replace it with another protein-rich food, such as fish or beans; cut milk out of your diet, and you can replace it with calcium-fortified soymilk.

Being able to include all foods in your diet doesn't mean that you can eat as much as you like of all of them. Limit your intake of high-GI foods or foods that contain a lot of fat.

Avoid diets that tell you to eat only organic or avoid any packaged foods. Because such diets can be costly and time-consuming (if you need to go out of your way to shop for organic foods), you may be less likely to stick to them. To date, no proof exists that organic food is more nutritious. The chemicals that are used to treat crops or in packaging materials have been tested and found to be safe at the levels that most people consume. However, if your budget can afford organic and you have strong convictions about this issue, eating organic can't hurt you as long as you're still getting a nutritionally balanced diet.

It Lets You Eat Only a Few Foods

Some diets work on the principle that they *bore* the weight off you! In other words, if they restrict your intake and allow you to eat only certain foods, you're unlikely to overeat. This goes beyond cutting out certain foods or a particular food group — this is restriction with a capital *R!* For example, such diets restrict what types of food you can eat from the various food groups (such as bananas from fruit, tuna from protein, and so on), or tell you to eat certain things on certain days (such as only meat on one day, and then all the vegetables you can eat on another day, but never combining meat and vegetables in a meal).

You'll find sticking to such a diet for longer than a week very hard, because you start to have strong urges to eat the foods that you're not allowed. Also, you may never want to eat the foods that you're allowed again, even if it's an ice cream diet!

The best sort of diet is a varied one. As a general rule, you need to have a variety of foods from each food group (refer to Table 14-1).

Doctors and dietitians do sometimes use a "few food diet" and a "rotation diet" made up of a few foods, in which individual foods are slowly added back in, but these diets are used under supervision to help identify particular food allergies. They aren't for weight loss.

It's High in One Particular Food Element

Good and bad foods don't exist — only good and bad diets. However, some foods can be eaten in larger quantities than others. Such foods include vegetables, fruits, and whole-grain cereals. Foods that can be included in the diet, but only in smaller amounts, include chocolate, cheese, nuts, butter, spreads, and oil.

However, if one food — no matter how "healthy" — is eaten to excess, it means that less room is available in your diet to eat a whole variety of other foods. Also, some foods may be high in certain nutrients, which if eaten in excess can lead to unwelcome consequences, some of which can be dangerous (see Table 14-2).

Table 14-2	What Can Happen If You Overconsume Certain Foods
Food	*Consequence of Overconsumption*
Liver	Vitamin A poisoning
Carrots	Skin can turn orange; vitamin A poisoning
Rhubarb	May reduce calcium absorption
Spinach	May reduce calcium absorption
Tea	Can reduce iron absorption
Milk	Can reduce iron absorption
Egg whites	Can inhibit the absorption of the B vitamin biotin
Bran	Can reduce the absorption of several minerals, including iron
Legumes	Can reduce the absorption of several minerals, including iron

It Has Too Much Protein Power (Combined with Low Carbs)

Some diets, such as the Atkins diet, suggest that you increase the amount of protein that you eat. Low-carbohydrate/high-protein diets seem attractive to many people because they set no limit on the amount of certain types of foods you can eat, may reduce hunger and appetite, and, at times, produce steady weight loss, even after failure or weight gain on other diets. However a high-protein diet is not a good idea for a number of reasons:

✔ **High-protein foods are likely to be high in cholesterol and saturated fats** — substances that can promote heart disease and various cancers.

✔ **In the absence of carbohydrate fuel, your body is forced to burn fat and protein to fulfill its energy needs.** *Ketones* (the breakdown products of burning large quantities of body fat for fuel) begin to accumulate in your body. A buildup of ketones in the body can cause all kinds of damage to your vital organs, such as the liver and kidneys. The buildup throws off your body's balance of acids and alkalines, causing a condition called *acidosis*. When the levels of ketones in your body reach dangerous proportions, you may slip into a coma, which can result in death. This is more likely to happen if you're a diabetic who has high glucose levels than it is from following an Atkins-type diet, however.

✔ **The accumulation of ketones in your body can leave you with unpleasant body odor and bad breath.**

✔ **You can lose muscle tissue as well as fat** — which is not the object of weight-loss diets. Ironically, the more carbohydrate you cut out of your diet and the more protein you eat, the lower your body protein stores become, because you're burning protein foods as fuel.

✔ **Not consuming a wide enough range of foods can lead to deficiency diseases.**

✔ **Cutting out carbohydrates can cause severe constipation.** Carbohydrates such as fruits, vegetables, and grains and cereals (particularly the whole-grain varieties) are the main source of dietary fiber. Eliminating these foods in the long run can lead to diverticulitis and irritable bowel syndrome, and it may even make you more susceptible to bowel cancer.

✔ **Consuming a lot of red meat is associated with an increased risk of colon cancer.**

✔ **Such a diet may exacerbate gout because it may lead to a buildup of uric acid in the blood.**

✔ **You may experience increases in serum triglycerides and low-density lipoprotein cholesterol,** both bad fats that can trigger heart disease — in particular blocked arteries and cardiac arrhythmias.

✔ **Such diets have been associated with *hypothyroidism* (low thyroid function).**

✔ **High-protein liquid diets have been associated with several sudden cardiac deaths due to severe electrolyte imbalances.**

✔ **Low-carb, high-protein diets shouldn't be coupled with a low calorie intake because this combination can trigger severe loss of important minerals to the body, which itself can trigger sudden cardiac death.**

Blood cholesterol, sugar, and triglycerides may be reduced on high-protein diets because you tend to eat much less due to loss of appetite and sometimes nausea. In general, weight loss and health benefits are temporary because the high-protein plan is too unpleasant to continue — so you may be tempted to return to your old way of eating.

It Relies on Taking a Supplement or a Particular Substance

Although the days of fast-fix diet pills, which were downright dangerous, are long gone, this hasn't stopped the snake-oil sellers from still trying to promote their wares. The new generation of substances claiming to aid weight loss are not usually very dangerous, but they tend to be a load of hype that may cost you lots of money and deliver nothing. Such diets often claim that you can continue eating as much as you like and still lose weight. Unfortunately, this just isn't the case.

Table 14-3 lists some common substances claiming special weight-loss benefits today.

Table 14-3	Substances That Claim They Aid Weight Loss
Substance	*What It Claims to Do*
Diuretics	Diuretics make you urinate more. So, all you lose is water weight. Unfortunately, the fat stays right where it is. As soon as you drink more fluid, the weight returns.
Herbals	Many herbals that claim to have brought about weight loss have now been banned. Some of these actually caused serious damage to the liver and kidneys. However, other herbals that are unlikely to aid weight loss are still on the market.
Calcium (from dairy products)	Some evidence exists that a high calcium intake from dairy products can boost metabolism. In fact, other dairy components may be having the active effect. However, even if high calcium intake does boost metabolism, it's doubtful that the amount is significant.
Green tea	Green tea and extracts of green tea are believed to boost metabolism. Again, the jury is out on this one.
Conjugated linoleic acid (CLA)	CLA is a naturally occurring fatty acid found in meat and dairy products. It's also a popular dietary supplement that is sold with claims of helping people lose fat, maintain weight loss, retain lean muscle mass, and control type 2 diabetes. However, CLA also may increase levels of bad fats in the bloodstream. More research is needed before CLA can be promoted as a risk-free and effective weight-loss aid.

Only taking in fewer calories than your body actually uses is going to lead to long-term weight loss. If your diet is balanced, and as long as you don't restrict your calorie intake below 1,500 calories per day, you shouldn't need to take any additional supplements because the diet provides you with all the vitamins and minerals your body needs. A diet that suggests that you also need to take vitamin and mineral supplements is probably advocating this because it's unbalanced and inadequate.

 The claims for many of these products are based on faulty and inadequate "studies." They aren't tested under rigorous scientific conditions; instead, these claims are based on small, uncontrolled "trials" that are set up to "prove" the claims. When most of these products and diets are subjected to truly rigorous, controlled studies, they show absolutely no benefit.

It Says You Have to Eat Loads of a Particular Food

Although it seems counterintuitive to be able to eat loads of a particular food when trying to lose weight, the thinking behind this sort of diet is that you only, or mainly, eat just one kind of product. If you can actually stick to the diet, you soon realize that there's a limit to how much of one food you can eat, so, of course, you lose weight in the short term. Not only is such a diet unbalanced, not providing all the nutrients that your body needs, but also you're unlikely to be able to stick to it for more than a few days.

Famous examples of this sort of diet included the cabbage soup diet, the grapefruit diet, and even the Mars bar diet. The cabbage soup diet, for example, claims that you can lose 10 pounds in seven days. For a start, this weight loss is not a safe, achievable goal in such a short period of time, and much of the weight loss is likely to be water. In addition to encouraging the eating of cabbage soup at least once a day, the diet (which should only be followed for seven days, but then what?) has you eating nothing but bananas, skim milk, and cabbage soup one day; just meat and tomatoes and, of course, cabbage soup another day; and so on. Although such a diet is meant to be a kick-start for a short period only, it isn't balanced, is too severe, and is likely to cause you to regain the weight when you stop. It also doesn't reprogram your eating habits for the better.

It's Very Low in Calories

The definition of a very low-calorie diet is a diet that provides only around 500 calories per day. Only people who are being closely monitored, such as in a hospital setting, should follow very low-calorie diets.

Many dangers of following a very low-calorie diet exist, but sometimes it's the lesser of two dangers — for example, in the case of a very overweight patient who needs a lifesaving operation but whose weight makes it a huge risk to have the operation unless she loses some weight. Such a diet should only be used in cases such as this, where rapid weight loss is imperative and the lesser risk.

Here are some reasons why you shouldn't put yourself on such a strict regime:

- **Side effects can include fatigue, constipation, nausea, and diarrhea.**

- **As you lower your caloric intake, getting all the nutrients you need from your food becomes increasingly difficult.** Lowering your diet to around 500 calories per day means that you're unlikely to get sufficient vitamins and minerals. You can take supplements, but these aren't guaranteed to provide you with the full range of nutrients and antioxidants, and their *bioavailability* (the ease with which they're absorbed into the bloodstream) isn't as strong as the bioavailability of real food.

- **These diets can lead to muscle loss as well as fat loss, which is extremely unhealthy.** To lose heart muscle, for example, is potentially fatal.

- **These diets don't change long-established bad eating patterns, and they cause the body to slow down significantly.** So, when you return to a more normal eating pattern, the lower metabolism may lead to increased weight gain.

It Has Strict Rules on What You Can and Can't Eat

If a diet comes with too many rules that shouldn't be broken in order for it to work, you're unlikely to be able to stick to it for very long. Nothing is more likely to make you crave certain foods than telling you not to eat them. Such diets also may restrict you *to* certain foods, which again is likely to lead to diet boredom and may mean your diet doesn't contain the full range of nutrients your body needs.

Good diets don't forbid you to eat certain foods, but they do indicate that you need to watch how *much* of certain foods you eat.
These foods include the following:

✔ Foods with a high glycemic index

✔ Foods that are high in fat (because they tend to be very high
in calories and also may contribute to developing heart disease and cancers), such as butter, spreads, oils, and pastries

✔ Foods that are high in a combination of fat and sugar (because
these tend to be calorie dense — you can't eat much of them
without racking up a high calorie count), such as chocolate,
candy, cakes, cookies, and pies

Foods that you can eat more freely include the following:

✔ Vegetables, including salad vegetables (but watch how much
high-fat dressing you use)

✔ Fruit, although overdoing fruit intake can make the calories
add up

✔ Beans, peas, and lentils

✔ Low-fat dairy products

What's important is the overall balance of the diet. You shouldn't
have to agonize too much about individual foods, but think more
about how they fit into your overall diet and how often and how
much of them you can eat.

Your Family and Friends Wouldn't Touch It

You don't want to have to become a recluse with your diet. Is your
diet the sort that none of your family and friends would eat? If it is,
why are *you* eating it?

Part of the pleasure of eating is to be sociable and to be able to
share the occasion with family and friends. Your diet shouldn't
exclude you from enjoying social occasions.

Don't forget that your new diet isn't something you're going to
follow for a week or two and then return to your usual habits. After
all, those usual habits got you into trouble in the first place! Your
new diet should be healthy and balanced, but it also should be
based on tasty foods that you, your family, and your friends can
equally enjoy.

Your diet also shouldn't be based on unusual foods that can be found only in specialty shops or that demand hours of preparation. Unless you become an obsessive-compulsive recluse, you aren't able to maintain such a diet.

You Can't Follow It for Life

Don't think of your PCOS diet as one you can go on for a while, and then return to your past eating habits. PCOS has no cure, but you can control it so that you can reduce the symptoms or, in many cases, reverse them altogether. But this result can be achieved only by permanently changing your eating habits and your life-style. So, whatever diet you follow has to be permanent.

Of course, you may need to cut the calories for a bit until you get to a normal weight, but the nature and balance of the diet needs to remain the same.

In order to see you through the rest of your life, a diet for PCOS needs to

✔ Be based mostly on low-GI carbs

✔ Be low in saturated fat and salt

✔ Not be too restrictive in calories

✔ Allow for three meals a day, plus some snacks

✔ Be based on normal, everyday food

✔ Be easy to make each meal

✔ Be forgiving if you occasionally slip up and splurge

Chapter 15

Ten PCOS Superfoods

In This Chapter

▶ Discovering foods that stand out from the crowd

▶ Identifying food properties that may help you with PCOS

▶ Challenging you to incorporate superfoods into your diet

Some foods and food groups fit in particularly well to the PCOS diet, and we highlight them in this chapter. You don't have to eat all these foods every day, but each one packs a lot of nutritional power, so try to find room for most of them during the course of a week.

Whole-Grain Breakfast Cereals

Diets that are rich in whole-grain foods have been shown to offer a number of health benefits. As far as PCOS is concerned, the main benefits are that whole grains are believed to lower insulin resistance and help control your weight. Experts now advise you to eat 16 grams of whole grains three times a day, for a total of 48 grams per day.

Whole grains are cereal grains that retain the *bran* (the outer layer) and the *germ* (the seed in the middle) as well as the *endosperm* (the starchy bit inside), in contrast to refined grains, which retain only the starchy endosperm. Whole-grain foods are those in which 51 percent or more of the ingredients consist of whole grains.

Whole-grain breakfast cereals are a great way to start the day for a number of reasons:

✔ They help to fill you up and stop you from feeling hungry too soon before lunch because they're rich in fiber, contain some protein, and have a low glycemic index (GI). (Turn to Chapter 4 for a complete explanation of the GI and how it affects your diet.)

✔ They provide essential fiber and lots of vitamins and minerals.

✔ They're low in fat.

Here are some examples of whole-grain breakfast cereals:

- ✔ Muesli or granola
- ✔ Oatmeal made with unprocessed oats
- ✔ Shredded Wheat
- ✔ Cheerios
- ✔ Raisin Bran
- ✔ Grape-Nuts

Whole-Wheat Pasta

Pasta is a great staple food because it has a low GI, is high in filling carbs, and provides lots of other nutrients. Pasta also tastes great and forms an excellent basis for many dishes. However, *whole-wheat* pasta is even better because, in addition having the properties of pasta, it also provides the following:

- ✔ **Fiber:** Whole-wheat pasta contains 4.5 grams of fiber per 100 grams, compared with 1.5 grams of fiber in regular pasta.

- ✔ **Vitamins and minerals,** including iron, selenium, magnesium, B vitamins, vitamin E, and phytochemicals that have antioxidant properties.

- ✔ **An even lower GI than regular pasta:** Whole-wheat pasta has a GI of 37, whereas regular pasta has a GI of 41. (Both values are classified as low.)

You may not always want to use whole-wheat pasta because some recipes lend themselves to the lighter, refined pasta, but experiment with different types of grains in pasta to see what works.

Whole-wheat pasta works particularly well if you're making soup, such as minestrone.

Sweet Potatoes

Sweet potatoes are as versatile as the humble spud, but for PCOS they have some advantages over ordinary potatoes. Sweet potatoes have a

- ✔ **Much lower GI than ordinary potatoes:** A baked sweet potato has a GI of 54, whereas an ordinary baked potato has a GI of 85.

   ✔ **Large amount of vitamins:** One baked sweet potato provides masses of beta-carotene, which the body converts into vitamin A. It's also a good source of vitamin C and a significant source of iron.

   ✔ **Rich orange color:** This means that sweet potatoes contain phytochemicals, which act as potent antioxidants in the body.

 In most recipes that use ordinary potatoes, you can substitute the ordinary potatoes in part or wholly with sweet potatoes, but keep in mind that sweet potatoes generally take less time to cook than ordinary potatoes do (five to ten minutes less). Sweet potatoes have a slightly sweet taste, which goes well with strong meat flavors and most veggie dishes but may not go so well with fish; a 50/50 mix with ordinary potato is preferable in fish dishes.

 Choose sweet potatoes of a deep orange color and store them in a dry environment. Don't put them in the fridge because temperatures below 55°F can chill this tropical vegetable, giving it a hard core and an undesirable taste.

Beans

Beans have all kinds of benefits, including the following:

   ✔ They're versatile and tasty.

   ✔ They have a very low GI.

   ✔ They're nutritious and high in fiber.

   ✔ They're a good source of protein.

   ✔ They're rich in antioxidants, such as isoflavones.

   ✔ They contain anti-cancer substances called lignans. (Friendly bacteria in the colon convert lignans into hormone-like substances, which scientists say may fight off breast and colon cancers.)

   ✔ They can help lower cholesterol levels.

   ✔ They count as a vegetable if you're trying to make sure you have at least five fruits and vegetables a day.

   ✔ They can help you keep away hunger for some hours after eating them due to their high fiber and low GI values. Along with their very low fat content, they may be able to help with weight loss.

Here's a list of some common beans you can easily buy; their GI values are in parentheses:

- ✔ Butter beans (31)

- ✔ Soybeans (18)

- ✔ Red kidney beans (27)

- ✔ Navy beans (38)

With so much going for them, why not eat beans all the time? Well, they do have one small drawback: They can produce gas. However, gas is usually more of a problem when you first introduce beans to your diet; as your digestive system gets used to the beans, this problem typically diminishes. Just don't start eating a bean dish right before that first hot date or big job interview.

Most beans come dried, and they have to be soaked and then boiled before eating. For red kidney beans, this boiling process is essential because it destroys a toxin in the bean that otherwise gives you a very nasty stomachache.

To save time and effort, you can buy most beans in cans, which are ready to use and don't require boiling or soaking. However, because of the processing they've undergone, the GI of canned beans, although still classified as low, is higher than that of beans you soak and boil yourself.

Some beans, such as fava beans and soybeans, can be eaten fresh. These beans can be a very nutritious vegetable side dish.

Lentils

Lentils are legumes and cousins to the pea. They can be cooked in many ways, as well as being ground into a flour. Lentils are a PCOS superfood because they're

- ✔ Rich in protein and carbohydrates and a good source of calcium, phosphorus, iron, and B vitamins

- ✔ Low in fat

- ✔ Versatile in recipes and particularly useful for filling out meat in a dish, contributing a low-fat source of protein

- ✔ A vegetable, so they count toward your five fruits and veggies a day

✔ High in soluble fiber, so they can help lower your cholesterol level

✔ Low GI (with an average GI of 27)

Many varieties of lentils are grown and eaten throughout the world, but the three most common types used in cooking are brown, red, and green.

Lentils don't require soaking. However, you can soak them for a few hours if you want to; this reduces the cooking time by about half. You can substitute one type of lentil for another, although you may need to adjust the cooking time.

Nuts and Seeds

Having been almost scorned for a long while because of their fat content, these little gems are now beginning to hog the limelight as far as health-giving properties are concerned.

Yes, nuts and seeds do contain oil, and their oils are often extracted to produce vegetable oils suitable for culinary uses such as salad dressings. However, the oil in nuts and seeds is predominantly monounsaturated and polyunsaturated, and they're a good source of omega-3s.

Because of their unique blend of oils, protein, low-GI properties, vitamins, minerals, and antioxidants, nuts and seeds are believed to be great for your heart and can help to normalize blood fats. A small handful each day may even help you to control your weight.

You can sprinkle nuts and seeds on salads or add them to breakfast cereals. You can incorporate them into breads, cakes, or other baked goods. They also can be made into nut or seed butters, and don't forget the traditional veggie nut roast. A small handful of nuts and seeds also makes a great low-GI snack, which can help keep away hunger until your next meal. You can roast them to give more flavor, but avoid adding salt.

Here are some examples of nuts you may want to try:

✔ **Peanuts:** High in protein and 50 percent oil; used to make low-GI peanut butter, but look for peanut butters that don't contain hydrogenated oil.

✔ **Almonds:** Ground up, they form the basis of marzipan and often are used to add a rich texture to baked goods and desserts.

- **Walnuts:** They tend to go rancid very quickly, so they need to be stored in the fridge or freezer.

- **Cashews.**

- **Pistachios.**

- **Pine nuts:** Vital in pesto sauce.

- **Pecans:** Tend to be used in ice creams and desserts.

- **Brazil nuts:** An excellent source of the antioxidant selenium, which often can be in short supply in today's diet.

Here are some examples of seeds worth trying:

- **Sunflower.**

- **Pumpkin.**

- **Sesame:** The paste is used to make tahini.

- **Linseed:** Particularly rich in omega-3 fats, but best ground up before consumption or they tend to pass right through. However, if eaten unground, they're a useful laxative!

You don't need to eat lots of nuts and seeds to get the benefit, because they're a concentrated source of nutrients including vitamins A and E; minerals such as calcium, iron, zinc, phosphorous, and potassium; and fiber. About ¼ cup is a sensible portion.

Berries

Berries really are superfoods straight from nature. You can pick them right from the garden or gather them from woods and hedgerows to discover how delicious berries are. The most popular berries are naturally sweet, and making them into a tasty treat doesn't require much effort: Just rinse and serve them for a healthy, easy snack or dessert.

Berries are a good source of vitamins and *phytochemicals* (components of fruits or vegetables that have antioxidants and other health properties when you eat them). For instance, cranberries and blueberries contain a substance that helps prevent or treat painful bladder infections. Blueberries, strawberries, and raspberries also contain powerful antioxidants, which may help to keep away heart disease and cancers.

Berries, especially blueberries and raspberries, also contain lutein, which is important for healthy vision. Hopefully, further research on the different phytochemicals found in berries will prove fruitful (pun intended!).

In addition to containing health-giving substances, berries are also a great source of other nutrients — vitamin C, calcium, magnesium, folic acid, and potassium. Furthermore, they're all very low in calories at around only 45 calories to 80 calories per cup, and they have a low GI. One cup of raspberries offers vitamin C and potassium for 64 delicious calories.

In addition to eating them for dessert with some yogurt or low-fat ice cream, berries are great added to your favorite breakfast cereal and go well in smoothies. They also can be added to baked goods, such as muffins. Keep a stock of frozen mixed berries in the freezer so you can eat them year-round.

Yogurt

What a godsend! You can use yogurt in both sweet and savory dishes and in smoothies. Yogurt is great health-wise because

- ✔ Low-fat yogurt is low in calories.

- ✔ Yogurt has a low GI (around 33), so it can bring down the overall GI of dishes to which it is added.

- ✔ Yogurt contains many nutrients, including calcium and riboflavin.

- ✔ Bio or live yogurt contains probiotic bacteria, which are increasingly believed to have unique health-giving properties, including aiding digestive health, offsetting thrush, and boosting the immune function.

Always have some low-fat yogurt as a standby in the fridge: It adds a creamy texture in sauces and can be added on top of your favorite fruit as an instant dessert (it goes particularly well with berries). A serving of low-fat fruit yogurt makes a great low-fat, low-GI, low-calorie instant snack.

Green Vegetables

Your mother always told you to eat your greens for a reason! Unfortunately, our consumption of green veggies is on the decline, especially veggies such as cabbage and sprouts. However, the cruciferous family of vegetables in particular needs a helping hand in being elevated to superfood stardom. Cruciferous vegetables include

- Broccoli
- Brussels sprouts
- Cabbages
- Cauliflower
- Chinese greens
- Kale
- Purple sprouting broccoli

Cruciferous vegetables have certain health-giving properties, including the reduction of coronary heart disease and cancers. These properties are thought to be because these vegetables contain substances called *glucosinolates* (sulfur-containing compounds that act as anti-cancer agents). They also contain phenolic compounds, which act as antioxidants. Cruciferous veggies also are rich in several nutrients, including magnesium, folate, and vitamin C. However, if you cook these vegetables for too long or keep them warm for a while, you destroy some of the nutrients.

Sardines

These tasty little fish, often deemed to be too humble to be of any importance, are an oily fish high in omega-3 oils and fat-soluble vitamins D and E. They're also a rich source of iron and make a good, and much cheaper, substitute for rump steaks! Because sardines are very small fish, heavy-metal contamination, which can affect large fish, is less likely.

The canned versions are great made into pâtés and served on toast. If you flake them up with their bones, which become quite soft when canned, they're packed with calcium and are great for bone health. Sardines also can be purchased fresh; fresh sardines are ideal for grilling on a barbecue and serving with some fresh bread and a salad.

Population studies have shown that people who eat diets high in omega-3s have a reduced risk of heart disease. In basic terms, fish-eating populations are less likely to die prematurely of coronary heart disease. Current recommendations are to have two fish meals per week. Oily fish are best because they're highest in omega-3 fatty acids.

Chapter 16

Ten Places to Go to Get Information and Support

*W*hen you have PCOS, tapping in to resources for the latest information and meeting other women who are dealing with the same issues can be lifesavers. In this chapter, we show you where to find up-to-date information on PCOS, along with organizations that maintain active and helpful support groups and forums that can put you in touch with other women with PCOS.

Quite a few organizations claim to help women with PCOS but when you delve deeper, you find that they just want to sell you supplements or claim radical cures by use of crystals or avoiding electromagnetic radiation. Sometimes it seems as if we haven't come very far in the last 200 years — even in the 21st century, people are still trying to peddle snake oil that they claim cures all your ills, based on no scientific evidence.

Take with a grain of salt any organization that offers radical cures or claims that all you have to do is take a pill or supplements. You may not be an expert, but common sense — and the advice in this book — can go a long way toward sorting out the good advice from the bad.

Polycystic Ovarian Syndrome Association

The Polycystic Ovarian Syndrome Association (www.pcosupport.org) provides comprehensive information, support, and advocacy for women and girls with PCOS. It offers up-to-date educational resources and information on medical, surgical, and alternative therapies, as well as lifestyle practices that may be beneficial to women with PCOS.

Other services it offers include the following:

- ✔ Support and advocacy resources for women with PCOS
- ✔ Web services, including online discussion forums
- ✔ An online newsletter called *PCOS Today* and other articles and information on PCOS
- ✔ Conferences and symposia
- ✔ Local chapters and support groups

WomensHealth.gov

This website (www.womenshealth.gov/faq/polycystic-ovary-syndrome.cfm) connects you to the Office on Women's Health (OWH), which is part of the federal government. The mission of OWH is to work to improve the health and well-being of women and girls through its innovative programs, by educating health professionals, and by motivating behavior change in consumers through the dissemination of health information.

OWH was established in 1991 within the U.S. Department of Health and Human Services (HHS). OWH coordinates the efforts of all the HHS agencies and offices involved in women's health.

The website has some basic information about PCOS, as well as some great links to lead you to other sites that can give you more detail about various aspects of PCOS.

The site also contains lots of information on a variety of women's health concerns beyond PCOS. If you type in a subject in the search engine, it provides you with the most recent information about the subject.

The American Congress of Obstetricians and Gynecologists

The American Congress of Obstetricians and Gynecologists (ACOG; www.acog.org) is a professional organization for medical personnel, so it doesn't host discussion groups or online forums, but it does have all the latest research and information relating to PCOS. Any news that pertains to women's health is detailed on the ACOG site, which contains many links to articles about PCOS.

The American Association of Clinical Endocrinologists

Because PCOS is a disorder that affects the hormones, many of the specialists in the field of PCOS are endocrinologists. The American Association of Clinical Endocrinologists (AACE) maintains a list of endocrinologists at www.aace.com/resources/memsearch. php, which might make your search for a medical practitioner with a special interest in treating PCOS easier.

SoulCysters

In addition to having a clever name, SoulCysters (www.soulcysters. com) serves up what the site claims is the largest online community and support group dealing with PCOS. Women who have PCOS themselves are often the best source of new information as well as the tips and tricks that make living with PCOS easier.

Discussion groups on SoulCysters focus on everything from general information about PCOS to new research and information on doctors and insurance issues. Infertility, different medications, diabetes, and all the other medical issues that can impact women with PCOS are also discussed. There's even a forum for discussing issues that come up when dealing with the man in your life.

iVillage

You can find a lot of down-to-earth information about PCOS based on current medical thinking on iVillage (www.ivillage.com).

You can become a member of iVillage for free and benefit from certain services, including a regular newsletter where you can specify which information you want to receive, so you don't have to read the horoscope and celebrity news iVillage offers, but you can opt for info on diet and fitness, women's health, and recipes.

Verity

Verity is one of the best-known U.K. charities for women whose lives are affected by PCOS. You can become a member of Verity for a small fee. You then receive an information pack, regular newsletters, and invitations to Verity conferences and events. And, of course, you're supporting Verity in its mission to share the truth about PCOS.

Verity invites real experts and doctors working in the field of PCOS to come along to the conferences, and you always have the opportunity to ask these experts questions. Transcripts of their talks are available on the Verity website (www.verity-pcos.org.uk). Verity has produced a number of fact sheets (free to members, for a fee to nonmembers). Verity's discussion board is available to members and nonmembers alike.

PubMed

PubMed (www.pubmed.gov) is a free website run by the U.S. National Library of Medicine. It publishes many *abstracts* (summaries of articles published in medical journals), along with some full-length articles. Find articles on PCOS simply by typing "PCOS" into the search bar and start reading through over 277,000 articles or abstracts on every type of study researchers have conducted on PCOS.

When reading through PubMed articles, be sure to check the date, because some articles are considerably out of date, having been originally published in the early 1930s or 1940s! You'd hate to get excited about a new, cutting-edge treatment only to find out it went out of fashion back in 1955.

Other PCOS Sufferers' Blogs

Sometimes other people with PCOS are among the best sources of information on what works, what doesn't, and which doctors are best at treating the condition. Reading other people's blogs can be fun and interesting as well as educational, as long as you don't believe everything you read. If someone's surefire way to treat PCOS sounds too good to be true, it probably is.

But at the same time, women who are living with the condition are highly motivated to seek out the best available treatments for themselves as well as for others, and they generally aren't interested in scamming anyone.

Finding PCOS blogs is as easy as typing "PCOS blog" into your favorite search engine. Blogs, by their nature, come and go frequently on the Internet, so don't be discouraged if the first few sites you try come up as "no longer available" or "site not found." There are many women out there pouring out their hearts and souls about PCOS and its effects on their lives, and reading their stories can help you feel better about your own struggles.

Your Medical Providers

Don't forget to tap into the knowledge base of your own medical providers when learning more about PCOS. If you've chosen a doctor who is truly interested in PCOS and stays current on the latest information, don't be shy about letting him or her know that you'd like all the latest cutting-edge information about this disease. Your doctor may be willing to photocopy pertinent articles from medical journals for you.

Index

• D •

BUSINESS, CAREERS & PERSONAL FINANCE

Accounting For Dummies, 4th Edition*
978-0-470-24600-9

Bookkeeping Workbook For Dummies†
978-0-470-16983-4

Commodities For Dummies
978-0-470-04928-0

Doing Business in China For Dummies
978-0-470-04929-7

E-Mail Marketing For Dummies
978-0-470-19087-6

Job Interviews For Dummies, 3rd Edition*†
978-0-470-17748-8

Personal Finance Workbook For Dummies*†
978-0-470-09933-9

Real Estate License Exams For Dummies
978-0-7645-7623-2

Six Sigma For Dummies
978-0-7645-6798-8

Small Business Kit For Dummies, 2nd Edition*†
978-0-7645-5984-6

Telephone Sales For Dummies
978-0-470-16836-3

BUSINESS PRODUCTIVITY & MICROSOFT OFFICE

Access 2007 For Dummies
978-0-470-03649-5

Excel 2007 For Dummies
978-0-470-03737-9

Office 2007 For Dummies
978-0-470-00923-9

Outlook 2007 For Dummies
978-0-470-03830-7

PowerPoint 2007 For Dummies
978-0-470-04059-1

Project 2007 For Dummies
978-0-470-03651-8

QuickBooks 2008 For Dummies
978-0-470-18470-7

Quicken 2008 For Dummies
978-0-470-17473-9

Salesforce.com For Dummies, 2nd Edition
978-0-470-04893-1

Word 2007 For Dummies
978-0-470-03658-7

EDUCATION, HISTORY, REFERENCE & TEST PREPARATION

African American History For Dummies
978-0-7645-5469-8

Algebra For Dummies
978-0-7645-5325-7

Algebra Workbook For Dummies
978-0-7645-8467-1

Art History For Dummies
978-0-470-09910-0

ASVAB For Dummies, 2nd Edition
978-0-470-10671-6

British Military History For Dummies
978-0-470-03213-8

Calculus For Dummies
978-0-7645-2498-1

Canadian History For Dummies, 2nd Edition
978-0-470-83656-9

Geometry Workbook For Dummies
978-0-471-79940-5

The SAT I For Dummies, 6th Edition
978-0-7645-7193-0

Series 7 Exam For Dummies
978-0-470-09932-2

World History For Dummies
978-0-7645-5242-7

FOOD, HOME, GARDEN, HOBBIES & HOME

Bridge For Dummies, 2nd Edition
978-0-471-92426-5

Coin Collecting For Dummies, 2nd Edition
978-0-470-22275-1

Cooking Basics For Dummies, 3rd Edition
978-0-7645-7206-7

Drawing For Dummies
978-0-7645-5476-6

Etiquette For Dummies, 2nd Edition
978-0-470-10672-3

Gardening Basics For Dummies*†
978-0-470-03749-2

Knitting Patterns For Dummies
978-0-470-04556-5

Living Gluten-Free For Dummies†
978-0-471-77383-2

Painting Do-It-Yourself For Dummies
978-0-470-17533-0

HEALTH, SELF HELP, PARENTING & PETS

Anger Management For Dummies
978-0-470-03715-7

Anxiety & Depression Workbook For Dummies
978-0-7645-9793-0

Dieting For Dummies, 2nd Edition
978-0-7645-4149-0

Dog Training For Dummies, 2nd Edition
978-0-7645-8418-3

Horseback Riding For Dummies
978-0-470-09719-9

Infertility For Dummies†
978-0-470-11518-3

Meditation For Dummies with CD-ROM, 2nd Edition
978-0-471-77774-8

Post-Traumatic Stress Disorder For Dummies
978-0-470-04922-8

Puppies For Dummies, 2nd Edition
978-0-470-03717-1

Thyroid For Dummies, 2nd Edition†
978-0-471-78755-6

Type 1 Diabetes For Dummies*†
978-0-470-17811-9

* Separate Canadian edition also available
† Separate U.K. edition also available

Available wherever books are sold. For more information or to order direct: U.S. customers visit www.dummies.com or call 1-877-762-2974. U.K. customers visit www.wileyeurope.com or call (0) 1243 843291. Canadian customers visit www.wiley.ca or call 1-800-567-4797.

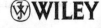

INTERNET & DIGITAL MEDIA

AdWords For Dummies
978-0-470-15252-2

Blogging For Dummies, 2nd Edition
978-0-470-23017-6

Digital Photography All-in-One Desk Reference For Dummies, 3rd Edition
978-0-470-03743-0

Digital Photography For Dummies, 5th Edition
978-0-7645-9802-9

Digital SLR Cameras & Photography For Dummies, 2nd Edition
978-0-470-14927-0

eBay Business All-in-One Desk Reference For Dummies
978-0-7645-8438-1

eBay For Dummies, 5th Edition*
978-0-470-04529-9

eBay Listings That Sell For Dummies
978-0-471-78912-3

Facebook For Dummies
978-0-470-26273-3

The Internet For Dummies, 11th Edition
978-0-470-12174-0

Investing Online For Dummies, 5th Edition
978-0-7645-8456-5

iPod & iTunes For Dummies, 5th Edition
978-0-470-17474-6

MySpace For Dummies
978-0-470-09529-4

Podcasting For Dummies
978-0-471-74898-4

Search Engine Optimization For Dummies, 2nd Edition
978-0-471-97998-2

Second Life For Dummies
978-0-470-18025-9

Starting an eBay Business For Dummies, 3rd Edition†
978-0-470-14924-9

GRAPHICS, DESIGN & WEB DEVELOPMENT

Adobe Creative Suite 3 Design Premium All-in-One Desk Reference For Dummies
978-0-470-11724-8

Adobe Web Suite CS3 All-in-One Desk Reference For Dummies
978-0-470-12099-6

AutoCAD 2008 For Dummies
978-0-470-11650-0

Building a Web Site For Dummies, 3rd Edition
978-0-470-14928-7

Creating Web Pages All-in-One Desk Reference For Dummies, 3rd Edition
978-0-470-09629-1

Creating Web Pages For Dummies, 8th Edition
978-0-470-08030-6

Dreamweaver CS3 For Dummies
978-0-470-11490-2

Flash CS3 For Dummies
978-0-470-12100-9

Google SketchUp For Dummies
978-0-470-13744-4

InDesign CS3 For Dummies
978-0-470-11865-8

Photoshop CS3 All-in-One Desk Reference For Dummies
978-0-470-11195-6

Photoshop CS3 For Dummies
978-0-470-11193-2

Photoshop Elements 5 For Dummies
978-0-470-09810-3

SolidWorks For Dummies
978-0-7645-9555-4

Visio 2007 For Dummies
978-0-470-08983-5

Web Design For Dummies, 2nd Edition
978-0-471-78117-2

Web Sites Do-It-Yourself For Dummies
978-0-470-16903-2

Web Stores Do-It-Yourself For Dummies
978-0-470-17443-2

LANGUAGES, RELIGION & SPIRITUALITY

Arabic For Dummies
978-0-471-77270-5

Chinese For Dummies, Audio Set
978-0-470-12766-7

French For Dummies
978-0-7645-5193-2

German For Dummies
978-0-7645-5195-6

Hebrew For Dummies
978-0-7645-5489-6

Ingles Para Dummies
978-0-7645-5427-8

Italian For Dummies, Audio Set
978-0-470-09586-7

Italian Verbs For Dummies
978-0-471-77389-4

Japanese For Dummies
978-0-7645-5429-2

Latin For Dummies
978-0-7645-5431-5

Portuguese For Dummies
978-0-471-78738-9

Russian For Dummies
978-0-471-78001-4

Spanish Phrases For Dummies
978-0-7645-7204-3

Spanish For Dummies
978-0-7645-5194-9

Spanish For Dummies, Audio Set
978-0-470-09585-0

The Bible For Dummies
978-0-7645-5296-0

Catholicism For Dummies
978-0-7645-5391-2

The Historical Jesus For Dummies
978-0-470-16785-4

Islam For Dummies
978-0-7645-5503-9

Spirituality For Dummies, 2nd Edition
978-0-470-19142-2

NETWORKING AND PROGRAMMING

ASP.NET 3.5 For Dummies
978-0-470-19592-5

C# 2008 For Dummies
978-0-470-19109-5

Hacking For Dummies, 2nd Edition
978-0-470-05235-8

Home Networking For Dummies, 4th Edition
978-0-470-11806-1

Java For Dummies, 4th Edition
978-0-470-08716-9

Microsoft® SQL Server™ 2008 All-in-One Desk Reference For Dummies
978-0-470-17954-3

Networking All-in-One Desk Reference For Dummies, 2nd Edition
978-0-7645-9939-2

Networking For Dummies, 8th Edition
978-0-470-05620-2

SharePoint 2007 For Dummies
978-0-470-09941-4

Wireless Home Networking For Dummies, 2nd Edition
978-0-471-74940-0

OPERATING SYSTEMS & COMPUTER BASICS

Mac For Dummies, 5th Edition
978-0-7645-8458-9

Laptops For Dummies, 2nd Edition
978-0-470-05432-1

Linux For Dummies, 8th Edition
978-0-470-11649-4

MacBook For Dummies
978-0-470-04859-7

**Mac OS X Leopard All-in-One
Desk Reference For Dummies**
978-0-470-05434-5

Mac OS X Leopard For Dummies
978-0-470-05433-8

Macs For Dummies, 9th Edition
978-0-470-04849-8

PCs For Dummies, 11th Edition
978-0-470-13728-4

Windows® Home Server For Dummies
978-0-470-18592-6

Windows Server 2008 For Dummies
978-0-470-18043-3

**Windows Vista All-in-One
Desk Reference For Dummies**
978-0-471-74941-7

Windows Vista For Dummies
978-0-471-75421-3

**Windows Vista Security
For Dummies**
978-0-470-11805-4

SPORTS, FITNESS & MUSIC

Coaching Hockey For Dummies
978-0-470-83685-9

Coaching Soccer For Dummies
978-0-471-77381-8

Fitness For Dummies, 3rd Edition
978-0-7645-7851-9

Football For Dummies, 3rd Edition
978-0-470-12536-6

GarageBand For Dummies
978-0-7645-7323-1

Golf For Dummies, 3rd Edition
978-0-471-76871-5

Guitar For Dummies, 2nd Edition
978-0-7645-9904-0

**Home Recording For Musicians
For Dummies, 2nd Edition**
978-0-7645-8884-6

**iPod & iTunes For Dummies,
5th Edition**
978-0-470-17474-6

Music Theory For Dummies
978-0-7645-7838-0

Stretching For Dummies
978-0-470-06741-3

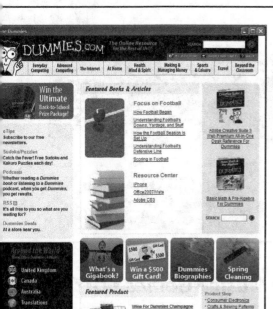

Get smart @ dummies.com®

- Find a full list of Dummies titles
- Look into loads of FREE on-site articles
- Sign up for FREE eTips e-mailed to you weekly
- See what other products carry the Dummies name
- Shop directly from the Dummies bookstore
- Enter to win new prizes every month!

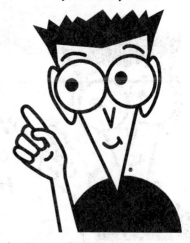

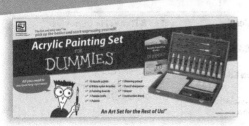
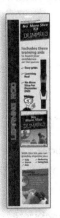
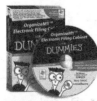
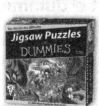
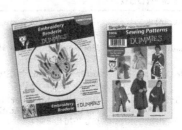
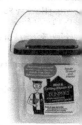

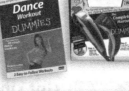
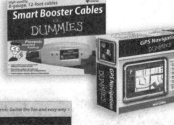
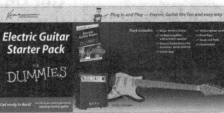
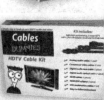

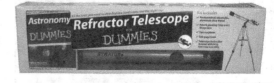
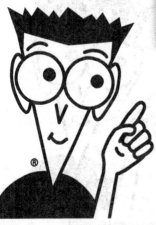